SMOKING AND CANCER

SMOKING

AND

CANCER

A Doctor's Report

By

ALTON OCHSNER, M.D.

JULIAN MESSNER, INC. • NEW YORK

Published by Julian Messner, Inc.
8 West 40th Street, New York 18

Copyright 1954, by Julian Messner, Inc.

Published simultaneously in Canada
by the Copp Clark Company, Ltd.

Library of Congress Catalog Card No. 54-10976

PRINTED IN THE UNITED STATES OF AMERICA

CONTENTS

Foreword by Evarts A. Graham, M.D.   vii

1. Smoker's Choice   1
2. Massive Proof by the American Cancer Society   4
3. What We Know About Cancer Incriminates Smoking   9
4. What Statistical Studies Have Proved   13
5. Smoked Mice and Smoking Men   20
6. Smoking and Sex   25
7. Cigars and Pipes and Respiratory Cancer   30
8. Smoking: Deadly Accomplice of Heart Disease   35
9. The King—and You   40
10. More Counts in the Indictment   46
11. Other Causes of Lung Cancer   50
12. Filters: A Help or a Hoax?   54
13. You *Can* Stop Smoking   57
14. How Smokers Can Minimize Their Health Risks   64
15. The Responsibility of the Industry   68
16. Cancer Can Be Conquered   76

References   83

Index   85

For permission to quote statistics and to reproduce the charts and graphs in this book, appreciation is expressed to:

The American Cancer Society
Journal of the American Medical Association
British Medical Journal
Journal of Cancer
Connecticut State Medical Journal
Archives of Industrial Hygiene & Occupational Medicine

Deep appreciation is also extended to the many scientists whose years of labor produced the conclusions expressed in this book.

FOREWORD

I am glad to have the opportunity to write a Foreword to this book by my friend, Dr. Ochsner. The subject is of major importance and any additional education of the public is to be welcomed.

Never before has it occurred that one type of cancer within a generation has moved up from a position of rare incidence to first place. But that has happened with lung cancer. Indeed only thirty years ago most doctors had never seen a case of primary cancer of the lung. Now, however, within the last two or three years it has superseded cancer of the stomach, which formerly occupied first place in incidence in men, to become the most frequent cancer in the male sex. This remarkable increase holds not only for the United States but for the western European countries as well.

Fortunately as the result of a large amount of research it is now possible to state that the chief factor responsible for this astounding increase has been the development of excessive cigarette smoking. Dr. Ochsner has given a good summary of the evidence for this point of view. Unfortunately it has not been universally accepted and there are still many cigarette addicts among the medical profession who demand absolute proof. However, the sort of proof which these die-hards demand would require human experimentation of a type which is impossible to consider. The obstinacy of many of them in refusing to accept the existing evidence compels me to conclude that it is their own addiction to this drug habit which blinds them. They have eyes to see but they see not because of their unwillingness or inability to give up smoking. On the other hand, if the evidence incriminated only an article of diet, such as spinach for example, probably nearly everybody would accept it as conclusive. I have never encountered any non-smoker who makes light of the evidence or is skeptical of the association between excessive cigarette smoking and lung cancer.

Of great importance is the realization that fourteen different statistical studies in three different countries have all shown the same result. There is no published study which shows a lack of association between lung cancer and excessive use of cigarettes. Is not this finding in itself significant? Probably it is important to distinguish between the use of tobacco and cigarette smoking. It is doubtful if they are synonymous. Many things are added to cigarettes, including paper, and nothing is known about the possible cancer-producing abilities of the combustion products of those substances. Moreover the curing and preparing of the tobacco used in cigarettes is different from the processes used for cigar and pipe tobacco.

All of this leads up to the question of what is going to be done about it. I am very glad that Dr. Ochsner has dealt with this question in his customary forthright and courageous manner. Are the manufacturers of cigarettes going to be allowed indefinitely to go on making addicts for their own profit by their alluring advertising? Are the radio and television networks to be permitted to continue carrying the advertising material of the cigarette industry? Isn't it time that the official guardian of the people's health, the United States Public Health Service, at least make a statement of warning?

EVARTS A. GRAHAM, M.D.

SMOKING AND CANCER

SMOKER'S CHOICE

CIGARETTES CAUSE CANCER.

Some of the most eminent scientists in the world believe that to be the fact.

Every type of smoking carries a deadly risk. Tobacco is a loaded, often lethal, weapon. Time pulls the trigger.

Medical leaders have battled to alert cigarette addicts to their suicidal folly. Until lately their warnings have been ignored by smokers. These warnings are still ridiculed by the tobacco industry.

In 1954 some 23,000 Americans will die from lung cancer. In 1955 approximately 25,000 Americans will die from lung cancer. In 95 per cent of the cases death will be traceable to smoking.

But the mortality rates are only indications. The casualties of war—and we are at war with cancer—are the sick and the maimed, as well as the dead. Lung cancer is in flood, and the flood is rising. "More Americans today are dying of lung cancer than died of all types of cancer fifty years ago," reports the American Cancer Society.

Lung cancer necessitates drastic surgery. In only one out of three victims brought to the hospital will the cancer be localized sufficiently so that the cancerous lung can be removed. Of these 85 per cent will be dead within five years, most of them within two.

All the skills of modern medicine will be unable to accomplish more.

True, even if you are a heavy smoker, you may not die of cancer. You may die of heart disease. Or a circulatory ailment. Or cerebral hemorrhage.

Or you may go blind from nicotine amblyopia.

Certainly you will lose most of your sense of taste and smell. You will become progressively more nervous and irritable. Your

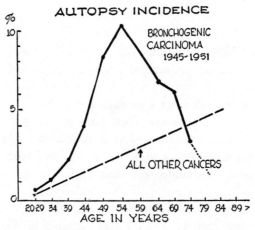

"Unless cigarette smokers die earlier from something else, they risk death from lung cancer about the age of fifty-five."

digestion will be bad. You will be troubled by one or more of such respiratory diseases as Smoker's Cough, Smoker's Throat, Smoker's Larynx, Smoker's Pharynx, Smoker's Asthma—familiar ailments directly traceable to smoking. There are even indications that if you are a man you may become impotent; if a woman, sterile.

This is the smoker's choice.

Unless you die earlier from something else, you risk death from lung cancer about the age of fifty-five.

This is no idle warning. The risks of getting lung cancer have been accurately calculated. The equation is simple:

The amount you have smoked daily and the number of years you have maintained the habit determine your chances of developing lung cancer.

A man of fifty who has smoked a pack of cigarettes a day for twenty years has fifty times more chance of contracting lung cancer than a non-smoker.

Research analysts describe a non-smoker as anybody who has not regularly smoked one cigarette per day for twenty years. A light smoker is one who has consumed from one to nine cigarettes a day for the same period. Smoking from ten to fifteen cigarettes daily makes one a moderately heavy smoker, and if one has smoked from sixteen to twenty a day for twenty years, he is a heavy smoker. An excessive smoker consumes from twenty-one to twenty-four cigarettes a day. More than that makes him a chain smoker.

Susceptibility, no doubt, plays a role in cancer. Less smoking may delay the onset of cancer; more smoking may hasten it. You may be able to take more tobacco abuse than others. But the definite relationship now established is that the more you smoke and the longer you smoke, the greater the risk.

Smoke unrestrainedly, and you probably advance your own death day.

MASSIVE PROOF BY THE
AMERICAN CANCER SOCIETY

IF THE CONCLUSIONS IN THE PRECEDING CHAPTER SEEM GRIM
and frightening, so is the problem which they deal with. Cancer
of the lung is a pandemic disease here and in northern Europe;
pandemic means widely epidemic. The death rate for respiratory
cancer of white males in the United States was six times greater
in 1953 than in 1930. The rise in lung cancer incidence has been
so awesome that "it is almost as though the population had been
exposed to some new hazard," Dr. Charles S. Cameron has stated
for the American Cancer Society. Death statistics show that in
1920 lung cancer caused 1.1 of every 100,000 deaths. In 1948
the lung-cancer deaths rose to 8.3 per 100,000. I predict that
in 1970, unless preventive measures are taken, lung cancer will
account for 18 per cent of all cancer deaths. This means that
one out of every ten to fifteen men who die in this country in
1970 will die from lung cancer.

Man is the only animal that pollutes his bodily structure by
smoking, and nature is teaching him a merciless lesson.

Notwithstanding the accumulation of clinical, statistical, and
laboratory findings pointing to tobacco as the lurking killer in
cancer and heart diseases, many still await the miracle of irrefutable scientific proof—the isolation of the carcinogen or carcinogens in tobacco smoke, from something like 200 chemical substances contained in tobacco tars alone. Proof, by some grisly
experiment on human beings, that what produces cancer in

animals can produce cancer in man! The world might have remained in a sorry plight for many years if British sanitarians waited for the discovery of the typhoid germ before accepting clinical and statistical evidence that certain wells in London were the real disease spreaders.

Proof has been piled upon proof associating the effects of compulsive smoking with cancer, with heart disease, with general respiratory and other diseases, only to strike a wall of medical skepticism at the outset.

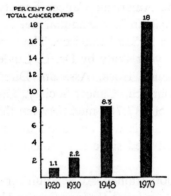

"One out of every ten to fifteen men who die in this country in 1970 will die from lung cancer."

With honorable exceptions, of course. The distinguished *New England Journal of Medicine* found that the evidence associating smoking and cancer must be considered "proof within the ordinary meaning of the word." So did the *British Medical Journal*— the voice of the British Medical Association.

"Statistics," it declared, "cannot prove causation. But neither could Koch's postulates, although the lives of millions are affected and controlled on the assumption that they have established beyond question the causative agents of certain infective diseases."

It is natural that there should be some difference of opinion between non-smoking and smoking doctors. Dr. Walter C. Alvarez, consultant in medicine to the Mayo Clinic, has recently written in his popular medical column: "I remember some of my close friends in the medical profession, highly intelligent men, who knew all the dangers of the excessive use of tobacco and yet they went on with their chain smoking until, in their early fifties, they dropped dead with a coronary attack." If they hadn't, lung cancer probably would have got them.

For most of the medical profession, however, serious debate about cigarette smoking as a factor associated with an increase in the general death rate ended on June 21, 1954.

On that day, the American Cancer Society submitted a research report to physicians at the annual meeting of the American Medical Association in San Francisco. The report was the result of a two-and-a-half year study by Dr. E. Cuyler Hammond, Director, and Dr. Daniel Horn, Assistant Director of Statistical Research for the American Cancer Society. The study dealt with the smoking habits of 187,766 men between the ages of fifty and seventy, and the analysis was based on the reported deaths of 4,854 men who had died since the project was begun in January 1952.

More than 22,000 trained ACS volunteers were used. The survey covered 394 counties throughout the United States. And Dr. Charles S. Cameron, Medical and Scientific Director of the American Cancer Society, found the information "so clearly valid —beyond any question of statistical error," that it appeared to warrant publication before the time planned. The publication was advanced "to save lives," Dr. Hammond declared.

Point by point the American Cancer Society study—the first of its kind in history—confirmed the medical studies previously made and pushed ahead to new ground.

The over-all finding of the Hammond-Horn report, which struck the headlines with bomblike effect, was that cigarette smokers die sooner than other men in the fifty-to-seventy age bracket and that they die mainly from cancer and heart disease.

What many lay analysts failed to underscore is the profound importance to the American health community and the American public of the long-term trends with regard to smoking and health.

LUNG & BRONCHUS CANCER DEATH RATES, BY AGE & SEX
White Population of the United States, 1933-1936 and 1945-1948

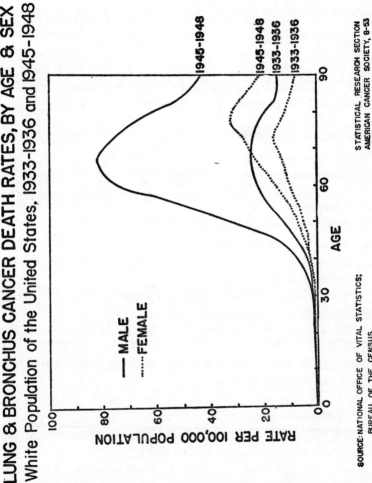

SOURCE: NATIONAL OFFICE OF VITAL STATISTICS;
BUREAU OF THE CENSUS

STATISTICAL RESEARCH SECTION
AMERICAN CANCER SOCIETY, 8-53

It is sufficient to quote Dr. Hammond's own words in his pre-publication report to the Board of Directors of the American Cancer Society.

1. *"Cigarette smoking is associated with an increase of the general death rate."*

Of the 4,854 men who had died, a total of 3,022 deaths occurred among regular cigarette smokers. If their death rates had been the same as for non-smokers, only 1,980 would have died.

2. *"Even light cigarette smoking is associated with increasing death rates."*

Death rates were appreciably higher among light cigarette smokers than among men who never smoked.

3. *"Cigarette smoking is associated with an increase in the death rate from most of the more common sites of cancer in men."*

A little less than half of the total increase observed was attributed to lung carcinoma.

4. *"Heavy smoking nearly doubles the death rate from diseases of the coronary arteries."*

It is almost two times as high among heavy smokers as among non-smokers.

5. *"Heavy cigarette smoking more than doubles the death rate from cancer."*

The cancer death rate was almost two and one half times as high as among non-smokers.

6. *"The findings were essentially the same for rural areas as well as for urban areas."*

Los Angeles, Chicago, Buffalo, Detroit, Minneapolis, and other centers were included in this survey.

7. *"The findings were based on the study of all other available experimental as well as statistical evidence bearing on the subject."*

On this basis Dr. Hammond found not merely "an association between cigarette smoking and death rates," but "a cause-and-effect relationship."

3

WHAT WE KNOW ABOUT CANCER INCRIMINATES SMOKING

IT IS GENERALLY AGREED THAT MOST CANCERS ARE CAUSED BY an irritant. These irritants are called carcinogens. Many of them are known, and undoubtedly hundreds more will be identified before the cancer riddle is eventually solved. Carcinogens usually enter the body from the outside and settle in the first vulnerable area. Then they begin a persistent irritation that gradually breaks down the normal body cell machinery.

In our present ignorance we do not know exactly what happens during this process. It appears, however, that when the normal machinery is sufficiently disturbed, a wild, uncontrollable cellular growth occurs. Whether these frantic cells become cancerous or whether the cancer cell is a parasitic cell already in the body and allowed to flourish under the adverse conditions created by the carcinogen has not been established.

Despite superficial differences in appearance, all cancer cells, wherever they are found in the body, possess physical features in common. The distinctive features of a cancer cell can be identified under the microscope in a test called a biopsy.

All cancer cells, however, are autonomous, in that nothing, at the present time, can stop their growth unless they are removed from the body by surgery or perhaps destroyed by X-ray or radium.

Cancer cells eat away the healthy tissues around them to make room for their own expansion. And cancer cells are invasive: entering the blood and lymph, they are carried throughout the body.

The original cancer growth is called the primary lesion, and various cancers take their names from the regions where they first appear.

A primary lesion of the lung is called bronchogenic carcinoma. From the primary lesion spread the secondaries—and there can be many of them. They are called metastases. The reason you are urged to be examined frequently—especially if you are a heavy smoker—is that, with luck, your doctor will detect the primary lesion before it metastasizes. The more metastases spread, the less can be done for you.

That the incessant use of tobacco is seriously irritating to the mucous membrane with which it comes in contact is no longer in question. That there is something in tobacco smoke capable of causing tissue changes in the respiratory tract is generally accepted. The *Journal of the American Medical Association* (March 29, 1952) has treated editorially Myerson's findings with regard to Smoker's Larynx—a diagnosis based on a history of excessive smoking and the appearance of one or more lesions on the vocal cords. Multiple tumor masses, covering both vocal cords, sometimes emerge in the later stages of the disease, requiring removal by surgical means.

More recently, the *Journal* (January 23, 1954) has commented on a separate clinical entity of the respiratory system, described by Waldbott, in which small lymphoid nodules form on the wall of the pharynx as the result of excessive smoking. In the early stages, states the *Journal,* a seven-day cure is the elimination of smoking. Advanced cases demand extensive antibiotic treatment, in addition to the avoidance of tobacco smoke.

My own suspicions about smoking were aroused some twenty years ago when I observed that most of the patients on whom I operated for ailments of the lung, heart, arteries, and stomach were heavy smokers. In medicine, when a single factor appears often enough in a wide number of cases, it assumes a significant importance.

I also observed that serious postoperative complications appeared most often among heavy smokers, less among light smokers, and rarely among non-smokers.

DEATH RATES FOR SELECTED RESPIRATORY DISEASES AND SITES OF CANCER AMONG WHITE MALES, United States, 1933-1948

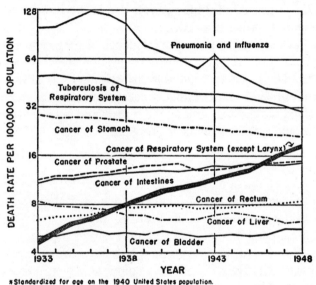

×Standardized for age on the 1940 United States population.

SOURCE: NATIONAL OFFICE OF VITAL STATISTICS

STATISTICAL RESEARCH SECTION
AMERICAN CANCER SOCIETY. 9-53

"Lung cancer deaths soared 144 per cent from 1939 to 1949. All other types of cancer deaths rose only 31 per cent."

With the aid of my staff I looked further into these situations and discovered some startling facts. These facts hold up today:

The increase of lung-cancer deaths in the past twenty years has been in direct proportion to the increase of cigarette sales.

Of all the lung-cancer patients studied in hospitals in recent years, more than 95 per cent admit that they have been moderate to heavy smokers for long periods.

Lung cancer deaths soared 144 per cent from 1939 to 1949. All other types of cancer deaths rose only 31 per cent.

We found that the increase in cigarette consumption paralleled the increase in lung-cancer incidence. In 1930, for instance, 3,848 lung-cancer deaths were reported in the United States. In the same year, Americans smoked 123 billion cigarettes. Ten years later, in 1940, there were 9,543 reported deaths from lung cancer. The nation smoked 189 billion cigarettes.

In 1953, when 22,000 lung-cancer deaths were reported, 394 billion cigarettes were smoked.

Thus in twenty-three years the incidence of lung-cancer deaths rose 471 per cent, while cigarette consumption rose 220 per cent.

In 1912 Dr. I. Adler, a notable investigator, was able to find reports of only 374 cases of lung cancer in our medical literature. He classified the disease "among the rarest" and believed it would never become a serious medical problem.

During my own student days, a decade later, I saw only one lung-cancer case in four years.

Today I operate upon from two to five such cases every week.

With the accumulation of clinical and statistical experience, I have carefully recorded over the years my preoperative diagnosis. When I see a patient who clinically has symptoms of lung cancer and who presents at the same time a history of heavy smoking, I put it down tentatively that he has epidermoid lung cancer, the scaly or platelike squamous-cell cancer. Or what has become known as Smoker's Cancer. Thus far I have been right in 98 per cent of my diagnoses.

If the patient is a non-smoker I put it down, preoperatively, that it is a case of adenocarcinoma, a rare type of lung cancer not produced by smoking, or an inflammation. So far I have been right in 100 per cent of the cases, although sooner or later an exception is bound to occur.

It is not surprising, therefore, that the present American Cancer Society study concludes that heavy cigarette smoking more than doubles the death rate from cancer.

4

WHAT STATISTICAL STUDIES HAVE PROVED

THE CONTINUING STATISTICAL SURVEY OF THE AMERICAN Cancer Society, already referred to, has opened up new lines of inquiry with regard to the association of smoking with an increase in the death rate for most of the more common sites of cancer in men. For lung cancer, and other cancers of the respiratory tract, the definitive surveys to determine the relation of smoking to cancer were those conducted through medical studies of the smoking histories of hospitalized patients in the United States, England and elsewhere.

Among the most important of these studies was the 1950 Wynder-Graham report, covering 684 proven cases in men and women. Its authors were Professor Evarts A. Graham of Washington University, the eminent surgeon who, in 1933, performed the first successful operation in history for the removal of a cancerous lung, and Dr. E. L. Wynder, of the Memorial Center for Cancer and Allied Diseases of New York City. Professor Graham's patient still lives and is engaged in active medical practice. They discovered that of 605 male lung-cancer cases, 96.5 per cent had smoked at least half a pack of cigarettes per day for twenty years; it was rare to find, they reported, a lung-cancer victim who had not smoked excessively for years. Of the 605 cases in males only eight had been non-smokers. "Excessive and prolonged use of tobacco, especially cigarettes, seems to be an important factor in the induction of bronchogenic carcinoma," they concluded.*

Almost identical findings were reported in England by Dr. Richard Doll and Professor A. Bradford Hill, who undertook a similar survey for the British Medical Research Council. Their preliminary report issued in 1950 declared that, "Smoking is a factor, and an important factor, in the production of carcinoma (cancer) of the lung." Their report was concluded in 1952.

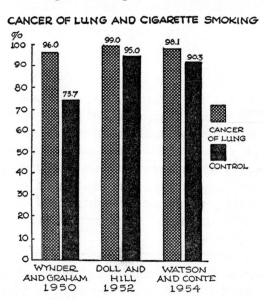

CANCER OF LUNG AND CIGARETTE SMOKING

Three separate surveys have resulted in almost identical findings.

Doll and Hill examined the case histories of 1,488 lung-cancer patients and compared them with 1,278 cases of cancer in other parts of the body and 1,465 cases involving diseases other than cancer. Among 1,357 men with lung cancer they found only seven who were non-smokers—half of 1 per cent. Among an equal number of patients with other diseases were 61 non-smok-

* The number of patients with proven cancer of the lung examined by Wynder and Graham was increased in 1951 to 857. The statistical results in the larger series were essentially the same as in the smaller series.

ers, 4.5 per cent. Statistically, this is a tremendously significant difference.

Taking into consideration the present smoking habits in London, Doll and Hill were able to deduce that of all the men in the

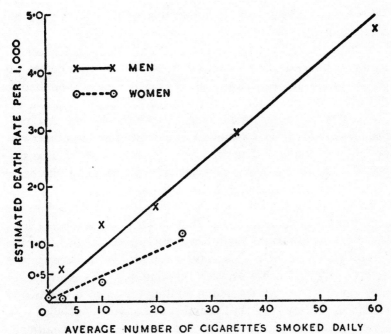

Estimated annual death rates from lung cancer in Greater London for men and for women aged 45–64, in relation to the average amount of tobacco smoked daily (measured in terms of cigarettes) in the preceding 10 years.

city from forty-five to sixty-four years of age, from three to five per 1,000 will die from lung cancer. The final report concluded that "the association between smoking and carcinoma of the lung is real"; that the risk of dying from lung cancer increases with age "and in approximately simple arithmetical proportion to the amount smoked."

The findings of every subsequent study have pointed relentlessly to a causal relationship of smoking to lung cancer. Dr. Herman E. Hilleboe, Commissioner of Health of New York State, where important lung-cancer researches have been conducted, states: "Well-designed and scientifically executed studies leave little doubt that a definite association exists between cigarette smoking and lung cancer," and that this relationship is probably a causal one.

Speaking as director of the Government's National Cancer Institute at Bethesda, Maryland, Dr. J. R. Heller, even before the publication of the American Cancer Society figures submitted to the 1954 convention of the American Medical Association, declared: "We agree that the evidence presently accumulated justifies the belief that heavy smokers of cigarettes are at greater risk of cancer of the lung than are non-smokers. . . . We will be surprised if the direct studies now under way, including one being initiated here, do not establish this belief as a fact."

In appraising the evidence that had piled up even before the report of the American Cancer Society, Dr. C. P. Rhoads, Director of the world-famous Sloan-Kettering Institute of the Memorial Cancer Center in New York City, declared: "We believe there is a very real relationship between smoking and the occurrence of lung cancer." A panel discussion on lung cancer by distinguished physicians in New York in December of last year concluded with this summary statement by Dr. Claude E. Forkner, chairman: "The risk of developing cancer of the lung increases in direct proportion to the amount smoked. It is rare for a non-smoker to develop cancer of the lung."

So impressive were the findings of the Doll-Hill report and subsequent studies by British cancer authorities that Ian Macleod, British Minister of Health, rose in the house of Commons early this year to warn British youth on the risks of smoking and lung cancer. He declared that he accepted the report of the British Committee on Cancer and Radiotherapy which concluded that "young people should be warned of the risks apparently attendant on excessive smoking."

Dr. J. G. Scadding, Director of Studies of the Institute of the Chest in England, in broadcasting to the nation the famous Doll-Hill findings, declared: "We can conclude that heavy smoking predisposes to lung cancer. The odds of a non-smoker dying of cancer in the next twelve months are 10,000 to 1. They shorten to 300 to 1 in the case of the heavy smoker."

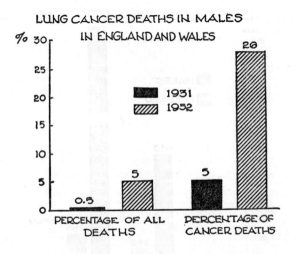

In France Dr. Oberling, Director of the National Research Center of the National Cancer Institute, accepts as conclusive the findings published in the United States and Great Britain that definitely associate smoking and cancer. No further evidence, he declares, is necessary to establish the cause-and-effect relationship.

Dr. R. Korteweg, leading Dutch cancer authority, has stated: "Before long in the Netherlands and in many other countries lung-cancer mortality will mount to from 25 per cent to 40 per cent of the total cancer mortality in males. Unless all indications are misleading, tobacco smoking is one of the important causes of lung cancer. . . . Failure to warn the public against the danger is no longer justified."

Nearly a 500 per cent rise in lung-cancer mortality has occurred in the last twenty years, paralleling the huge increase in cigarette consumption. Yet only a few years ago medical eyebrows were raised high at the suggestion that a causal relationship, not merely an association, had been established between

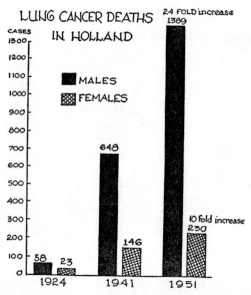

Lung cancer since 1924 has increased ten times in women and twenty-four times in men.

excessive cigarette smoking and the alarming increase in cancer of the lung.

In the study "Bronchogenic Carcinoma: Its Frequency, Diagnosis, and Early Treatment," by Drs. Alton Ochsner, Paul T. DeCamp, M. E. DeBakey, and C. J. Ray (*Journal of the American Medical Association,* March 1, 1952) we reported that "for some time two of us (Dr. DeBakey and the writer) have been convinced that there is a causal relationship between the increased incidence of bronchogenic carcinoma and the increased use of cigarettes." We showed that the annual production of cigarettes per capita population (including men, women, and children) increased from 46.3 in 1903 to 2,541 in 1948. From 1920 to 1930 the annual number of cigarettes per capita increased from 480 to 930; in the decade twenty years later, from 1938 to 1948, during which time the carcinogenic effect of the smoking in the earlier decade should have become evident. In the eighteen years from 1930 to 1948 the annual number of cigarettes per capita consumed jumped from 930 to 2,541 (2.6 times)."

By this time there is no longer any disposition among responsible cancer scientists to minimize the significance of these ominous statistical parallels. So great has been the shift of medical opinion that the recent Hammond-Horn report presented by the American Cancer Society does not hesitate to affirm a cause-and-effect relationship between smoking and cancer.

Indeed Dr. Horace Joules, Director of the Central Middlesex Hospital in London, finds in this statistical demonstration "one of the most important facts that has come to light concerning cancer during this century."

It has opened a new vista of cancer research for the clinician and the laboratory worker.

5

SMOKED MICE AND SMOKING MEN

ARMED WITH THE LATEST STATISTICAL EVIDENCE, RESEARCH scientists are exploring a thousand clues that may lead to the identification, isolation, and possible removal of the cancer-producing agent or agents still hidden in smoke. Already mice have helped to establish this much: The presence of a carcinogen in tobacco smoke.

This again was the achievement of Graham and Wynder, with Croninger as the research assistant. In Washington University, St. Louis, they constructed what looked like a small glass tree. In the branches were openings to hold cigarettes. By properly applying automatic suction, the scientists were able to simulate actual smoking conditions: the machine "puffed" on twenty-four burning cigarettes approximately three times a minute. The machine was so regulated that every eighteen seconds a "drag" of two seconds was taken.

The smoke was drawn into chilled flasks where it was condensed and tobacco tars were accumulated.

Taking the tobacco tar thus distilled from the actual cigarette smoke, the three scientists painted it on the shaved skin of mice. At first the tar was so potent that many of the mice promptly died from nicotine poisoning.

Then the tar was diluted and the skin painting performed three times a week. Even when diluted, the solution was so deadly that after a weekend layoff mice died with the Monday application. The solution was diluted still further.

After applying this milder solution for eight months, the scientists produced a tumor on one of the mice, but it proved to be non-cancerous. Four months later another mouse developed a tumor. It was cancer. Two years of steady painting with this solution was continued and cancers were produced on 44 per cent of the mice. And they were true cancers. This was proved by microscopic examination and by the fact that the cancers were transplantable within the mouse and to other mice.

None of the control mice (those not painted with the smoke residue) got cancer.

Skin cancers had been produced before by tobacco solutions. But this was the first experiment by which cancers had been produced at the site of application by tars obtained from cigarette smoke.

The presence of a carcinogen in cigarette *smoke* was categorically proven.

An earlier experiment with "smoked mice" conducted by Dr. J. N. Essenberg of the Chicago Medical School was not without significance. Dr. Essenberg sought to reproduce in mice the conditions to which human smokers subject themselves. He constructed two glass enclosures in which he placed mice that had been made cancer-susceptible by laboratory-controlled inbreeding and the frequent inducement of cancers in their ancestors. He attached to one of these enclosures a special device that "smoked" a cigarette an hour, sending the smoke to the mice inside. Mice in the second enclosure received ordinary air.

Of the twenty-three mice in the smoked-filled chamber, twenty-one had lung tumors within a year. Of the thirty-two mice in the smoke-free chamber, nineteen developed tumors within a year's time. None of these cancer-susceptible mice developed cancer of the type that excessive smoking produces in human beings. But what *was* proved is that smoking induces tissue changes that result in tumor formation.

As your cigarette burns, more than 200 chemical substances appear, flare up, and vanish. Many of them vanish down your throat, if you are a smoker. So much active chemistry occurs while you smoke that the greatest scientists have not yet figured it all out. Deadly poisons arise, rare compounds smoulder, elements unite. It's somewhat like puffing on a small H-bomb.

There are those who believe that what nature has put in tobacco man can remove so that smoking may become a less deadly diversion. They see great possibilities in the work now in progress here and abroad to discover and isolate the specific carcinogen or carcinogens still hidden in the poison maze of tobacco smoke. In the United States large-scale research is under way at the Institute of Industrial Medicine, part of New York University-Bellevue Medical Center in New York City, to identify the carcinogen, particularly in cigarette smoke.

The work is being carried on in this way:

All of the chemical compounds in tobacco smoke are being divided into eight groups, with as many as a dozen chemicals in each group. Solutions of the chemicals in each group are being painted on the mice. If the carcinogen in tobacco smoke is a single factor, then eventually only one group of mice will develop cancer.

The Institute scientists will then break down that group of compounds into smaller units and repeat the experiment, continuing in this way until the compounds are being applied singly to the mice. In that way the carcinogen or carcinogens will be isolated and identified.

None can estimate the time that will be required to identify the carcinogen by this necessarily laborious process.

Work at the Sloan-Kettering Institute in New York City has suggested that certain hydrocarbons in cigarette smoke may have much to do with lung cancer. Using the technique of the German scientist, Druckrey, the Sloan-Kettering Institute has been able to measure the amount of hydrocarbons that remain in the lungs when tobacco smoke is inhaled.

A puff of uninhaled tobacco smoke is released into a flask of pale liquid; a puff of inhaled smoke is released into a second flask. Exposed to ultra-violet rays, the liquids appear blue, but the flask containing the inhaled smoke is less opaque than the flask of un-inhaled smoke. This indicates that hydrocarbons of the inhaled smoke are retained in the lungs. Many doctors and laboratory workers who have witnessed the experiment have rushed to the nearest ash tray and given up cigarette smoking.

It could be that the cancer-producing factor eventually to be identified in tobacco smoke will prove to be benzpyrene, a known carcinogen found in coal tar and in the smoke of great cities. More than two decades ago Dr. H. Roffo in Buenos Aires concluded from clinical observations of some 78,000 patients that tobacco smoke was carcinogenic: he identified the carcinogen as benzpyrene. The Argentinian scientist wrote that with tars extracted from tobacco he was able to induce cancers on rabbits, both on the surface of the skin and in the lung. Later investigators, however, were not able to duplicate Roffo's experiments.

A clear and comprehensive summation of the facts that lead to the conclusion that there is a causal relationship between cigarette smoking and lung cancer was presented at the closing sessions of the Sixth International Cancer Congress held in São Paulo, Brazil, in July 1954. The main points were:

1. Cancer of the lung is rarely found in non-smokers.

2. Heavy smokers represent a much higher percentage of lung-cancer patients than of the general population.

3. There is a direct and recognized relationship between the amount smoked and the incidence of cancer.

4. There is a definite increase in the lung-cancer death rate in countries where there is a marked increase in tobacco consumption.

5. The increase in lung cancer is greater among men than women. Men frequently are heavier smokers.

6. The incidence of the disease is greater in cities than in the country, corresponding to greater cigarette consumption in metropolitan centers.

7. Most human lung cancers are of a type usually caused by irritants.

8. Similar cancers have been produced on the skin of animals by the application of the condensate from cigarette smoke.

9. Non-smokers who get lung cancers are those exposed to other irritants.

10. Lung cancer among non-smokers not exposed to other irritants generally is not the epidermoid type that smokers get.

6

SMOKING AND SEX

"BUT WHY DON'T WOMEN DIE FROM LUNG CANCER AT THE SAME rate as men? Look how they smoke!" This challenge is often hurled at cancer workers. I have my own answer. But the best answer may be: "Give them time and they will."

From four to five times as many men as women die from lung cancer. But the death rate in women is increasing. Recent statistics from Holland show that lung cancer since 1924 has increased ten times in women and twenty-four times in men. Women took up smoking during the 1920's and the habit became widespread after 1930; but they are still apprentice smokers compared to men.

Thus far the statistical studies of Wynder and Graham in this country and of Doll and Hill in England suggest that the greater mortality of men from lung cancer may be due merely to the fact that men have been smoking longer than women and tend to smoke more heavily. A statistical survey by Dr. Henry W. Ogden of the Louisiana State Medical School showed that males far outsmoke females; 60.2 per cent of males smoke compared to 26.4 per cent of females.

My own clinical experience leads me to believe that women smokers are less likely than men to develop lung cancer, possibly because the bronchial mucosa in women is less susceptible to malignant change than in men. However, we rarely see cancer of the lung in women and cancer of the lung in men who do not smoke. But almost without exception what we find in women is adenocarcinoma. This is a glandular cancer that develops from a congenital rest—possibly a remnant in the bronchial tube that has existed since the individual was born. The adenocarcinoma group is relatively small and with age the incidence of this form of lung cancer decreases, whereas with epidermoid cancer, re-

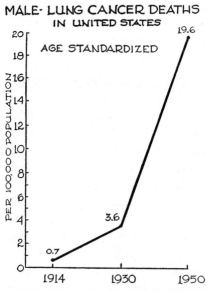

MALE-LUNG CANCER DEATHS
IN UNITED STATES

From four to five times as many men as women die from
lung cancer. . .

sulting mainly from tobacco as the extrinsic agent, the older the age group the greater the incidence of the disease.

We shall know more about the relative susceptibility of men and women to lung cancer when and if the cigarette industry consummates its progressive conquest of the feminine sex. But there seems little doubt that women are more sensitive than men in their response to nicotine specifically. Dr. Morris Friedell of the Hektoen Institute for Medical Research in Chicago has shown this by measuring changes in blood flow. Tests of fifty-two men, aged twenty-one to seventy and forty-eight women aged seventeen to sixty-one demonstrated that while smoking one cigarette the women averaged a 33 per cent change in blood volume as compared with 19 per cent in men. This, says Dr. Friedell, explains why women get a bigger "kick" from a cigarette than men, causing them to become more deeply addicted than men. Age, too, seems to make a difference. Many of the subjects over thirty-five, both men and women, showed no change in blood volume. This may be because the surface blood vessels of older persons are less sensitive.

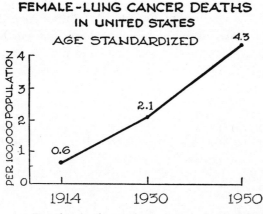

... But the death rate in women is increasing.

Writing in the *American Journal of Obstetrics and Gynecology* Dr. A. M. Campbell estimates that smoking has now become a significant factor in approximately 50 per cent of all obstetrical patients. He reports that smoking affects adversely the nervous system and the digestion, as well as the respiratory and circulatory systems, and that these adverse effects do not appear in the non-smoking obstetrical patients. Of the prominent obstetrical specialists questioned by Dr. Campbell, 96.9 per cent of those who replied agreed that the smoking and inhaling of twenty-five or more cigarettes a day would have an unfavorable effect on maternal health.

Repeated experiments have shown that nicotine is excreted in the milk and in the urine of all nursing mothers who smoke cigarettes. Dr. H. H. Perlman has shown that the amount of nicotine thus excreted correlates closely with the number of cigarettes smoked.

Sontag and Wallace have found that after an expectant mother smokes one cigarette there is an increase in the fetal heartbeat of five beats per minute. Dr. F. J. Shoeneck caused female rabbits to breathe cigarette smoke equivalent to twenty cigarettes a day smoked by a human being. Ten times as many baby rabbits were born dead from the mothers thus exposed, and the young that survived weighed 17 per cent less than normal.

With respect to reproduction, mice and men seem to be similarly affected. Essenberg reported that mice couples kept in his smoke chamber did not reproduce during the entire year they were subjected to cigarette smoke, while control mice continued to reproduce normally. He remarks that "the lack of reproduction among experimental animals is known to be caused by atrophic changes in the reproductive system. It is further known that the pathology caused by the injection of nicotine solution into mice or rats will parallel the pathology of the reproductive organs of mice exposed to cigarette smoke."

Other laboratory experiments have shown that female rats exposed to cigarette smoke suffer from temporary sterility and abortions; also that they average a disproportionate number of stillborn offspring.

Many physicians now agree that the decreased sexual activity of men in their thirties and forties can often be traced to excessive smoking. Dr. William Liebe has suggested that one reason for this may be that tobacco causes toxic changes in the blood which impede the formation of sexual hormones. Nor is this adverse effect confined to men. A German study of more than 5,000 women indicates that there may be a greater incidence of frigidity, sterility, menstrual disturbance, and miscarriage among women smokers than among non-smokers.

In England Dr. Lennox Johnston studied 500 men who had once been chain smokers but had discontinued smoking entirely. Their testimony is revealing at many points. The longer their continuance of the cigarette habit, the greater appeared to be the decline of sexual activity.

So firmly has the cigarette habit seized upon women that present estimates are that in the United States and Canada 59 per cent of all expectant mothers are now smokers.

There's point in the jibe that the first thing a modern child must learn in his mother's lap today is to watch out for the hot cigarette ashes from her burning fag.

7

CIGARS AND PIPES AND
RESPIRATORY CANCER

WHEN THE CONCLUDING REPORT OF DOLL AND HILL WAS BROAD-
cast in London in 1952, Dr. J. G. Scadding, Director of Studies
of the Institute of the Chest, who was in charge of the program,
told the people of England that he himself was sufficiently convinced by the evidence to have given up cigarette smoking in
favor of pipe smoking. "I would rather have a lip cancer that I
can see in time to cure it," he declared, "than a silent lung
cancer."

Nothing could better summarize the smoker's problem. It is
notable that Dr. E. Cuyler Hammond was equally convinced by
the American Cancer Society's study, a preliminary report of
which he submitted to the American Medical Association in June.
He, too, switched from cigarettes to a pipe. His study showed that
among smokers of pipes, cigars, or both, the death rate from all
forms of cancer is 32 per cent above that of non-smokers, whereas
among heavy cigarette smokers it is 156 per cent higher than
non-smokers, and 200 per cent higher for lung cancer.

Incessant smokers, for the most part, can choose the site of
their cancers. The cigarette smoker may prefer to risk cancer of
the lung; pipe smokers cancer of the lip; cigar smokers cancer of
the tongue. But the risk remains, and only a campaign of public
education can be expected to hammer this fact into the public
mind. General Ulysses S. Grant was perhaps the most inveterate

cigar smoker in the American Hall of Fame. The great military leader of the North had just forced the surrender of Fort Donelson, which commanded the river approach to Nashville, Tennessee. In the public mind his cigar-smoking habit was associated with his military prowess, and the General received a gift from his public of 11,000 cigars. General Grant died a tortured death from throat cancer. For months he had to sleep sitting up, while he heroically continued to write his military memoirs, undertaken after heavy financial losses had made his family penniless. He died four days after the completion of his work.

Most pipe smokers, it is true, consume less tobacco than cigarette smokers, which explains, in part, why they are less likely to get lung cancer. Heavy pipe smokers expose themselves to the same risks of lung cancer as heavy cigarette smokers. Doll and Hill found that of 1,350 lung-cancer patients, 3.9 per cent smoked pipes only. Of these, 9.4 per cent consumed the equivalent of only five cigarettes a day while 13 per cent smoked the equivalent of more than twenty-five cigarettes a day.

The Wynder-Graham study disclosed that American pipe smokers smoked more heavily than do Englishmen. In a study of 780 patients, 4 per cent were found to be pipe smokers exclusively and they daily consumed the equivalent of more than thirty-nine cigarettes. Such pipe addicts—a minority—are like cigarette chain smokers.

Drs. M. L. Levin, H. Goldstein, and P. R. Gerhardt reported in the *Journal of the American Medical Association*:

"Cancer of the lung occurs more than twice as frequently among those who have smoked cigarettes for twenty-five years than among other smokers or non-smokers of comparable age. Pipe smokers apparently experience an almost equal increase in the incidence of lip cancer, compared with other smokers or non-smokers."

The same research group found a parallel increase in tongue cancers among cigar smokers.

One cigar, according to evaluations by Graham and Wynder, is the equivalent of five cigarettes. Lung-cancer victims in the

Graham-Wynder study who smoked cigars exclusively consumed 6.9 cigars daily or the equivalent of approximately thirty-four cigarettes.

Dr. Wynder once said: "Frequently one is asked, 'What about Winston Churchill?' He certainly smokes heavily and is still free

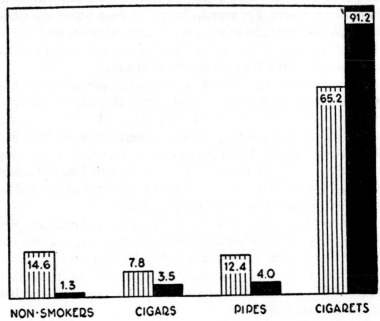

Smoking habits and type of tobacco smoked (in percentages) in 605 cases of lung cancer (solid bars) and 780 men in the general hospital population (lined bars) with a similar age and economic distribution.

of cancer. If we knew the answer to this question, we might have the answer to the cancer problem."

We can breed cancer-susceptible mice in the laboratory, but we do not understand the factors of predisposition that make some of the experimental animals cancer resistant and some susceptible. We do know, however, that tobacco is a factor in the production of lung cancer, and it is to the known factors that our preventive efforts must be directed.

The filtering qualities of pipes and cigars are easily recognizable: pipe smokers are well acquaintd with the soggy brown substances captured in the bowl and stem; similarly soggy brown butts are familiar to cigar smokers. Draw heavily while relighting a pipe or cigar and the tar-bitter elements enter your mouth. Recently a doctor painted the tar residue from pipes on laboratory mice: the animals died immediately. Even after the tar was weakened in solution, lesions appeared on the mice within two weeks.

This is the substance that men who chew tobacco or snuff bring into direct contact with their mouth tissues. At the University of Minnesota, Drs. George E. Moore, Lester L. Bissinger and Elsa C. Proehl found cancers in the mouths of twenty-six out of forty men who chewed tobacco. Eighteen out of another twenty-three who chewed had leukoplakia, a pre-cancerous condition of mouth sores.

In 1952 the production of chewing tobacco in the United States exceeded 40 million pounds; carcinoma of the oral cavity causes 4 per cent of the deaths attributable to cancer. In citing these figures, Greenberg, Lester, and Haggard remark: "Certainly if such a preventable circumstance as the chronic use of tobacco could be proved to be associated with the development of oral cancer, public education might result in a substantial decrease in these lesions."

Smokers who use pipes or cigarette holders complain of "tobacco bite." It is caused by the hot smoke that sears the same section of the tongue until irritation develops. The persistent combination of hot smoke and the concentrated deposits of nicotine and tars will cause cancer in the irritated zone as inevitably as will smoke in the lungs.

Smoke temperatures in cigarette holders can rise to 370 degrees when the butt is smoked too short. The faster you draw, the hotter the smoke. In pipes, the smoke can range in temperature from 550 to 1,200 degrees—several times the heat necessary to boil water at sea level.

No human tissue can take such punishment for any length of time. Cancer of lip, tongue, mouth, or larynx results.

Ordinarily, cigarette smokers hold the cigarette to their lips only when inhaling, and thus are less apt to develop cancers of the lip and mouth. This is not true of all cigarette smokers, however. One of my patients let a burning cigarette dangle constantly from the left side of his mouth while he worked. He developed cancer in the area. We removed it by surgery. For his own protection, I advised him to stop smoking, but, like so many smokers, he considered himself hopelessly addicted. In a futile gesture he transferred the cigarette to the right side of his mouth. In a short time he was back at the hospital; we removed a new cancer from the right side of his lip.

To a considerable extent you inhale whether you know it or not, regardless of whether you smoke cigarettes, pipes, or cigars.

Laboratory tests have shown that a quantity of tobacco smoke held in the mouth for a few seconds allows for a greater absorption of nicotine into the body than by actual inhalation. There is a possibility that this technique of smoking also permits tars to remain in the mouth longer than usual, and this would account for the increase in mouth cancers among pipe and cigar smokers.

Nonetheless, a certain amount of smoke, whether consciously inhaled or not, invariably reaches the lungs. It has been established that cancer growths among inhalers occur mostly in the peripheral regions; among non-inhalers the growth is most often in the central regions of the lung.

It is clear from all the data available that for the relentless smoker there is no escape in rushing from cigarette to pipe or to cigars. Like Drs. Scadding and Hammond, you can, by adopting a pipe, reduce the lethal risk of smoker's cancer—lung cancer. You can, more or less, choose the site of your cancer. You can choose the lesser risk—lip cancer or mouth cancer.

But since the smoking addiction is a breakable one you can also choose not to smoke at all.

8

SMOKING: DEADLY ACCOMPLICE OF HEART DISEASE

"HEAVY SMOKING NEARLY DOUBLES THE DEATH RATE FROM diseases of the coronary arteries." This, as will be recalled, was one of the major conclusions of the American Cancer Society's report, discussed earlier in this book.

Astonishing, startling were among the terms applied to the Hammond-Horn findings.

But considerably less "startled" was the medical profession, the great majority of whom here and abroad had for many years known of the association between smoking and heart disease. The report supplied overwhelming confirmation of what most doctors had long believed. It was, however, the first statistical proof of what clinicians had demonstrated by careful scientific experiments.

So extensive was the evidence that in its issue of November 8, 1952, the *Journal of the American Medical Association* noted editorially that the large majority of normal persons respond to cigarette smoking with definite peripheral vaso-constriction and warned that "although it may be generally concluded that cigarette smoking is most likely a contributory factor and not primarily an etiological (causative) one in the production of cardiovascular disease, physicians should pay more attention medically and pharmacologically to a nicotine-containing agent that is used by the public to an equal if not a greater extent than any drug."

Heart disease is not just one disease, but a collection of many diseases, with high blood pressure and coronary cases comprising two thirds of the total. It kills 52 per cent of our people. In 1953 more than 800,000 Americans died of heart ailments.

Sir William Osler, called the most beloved physician since Luke, said forty years ago: "Diseases of the coronary arteries and arteriosclerosis are frequently complicated by the use of tobacco." Little attention was paid to his warning. Today Dr. Irving S. Wright, Professor of Clinical Medicine at Cornell University, and recent President of the American Heart Association, declares that "The use of tobacco may mean the difference between life and death for persons with diseases of the circulation."

When I was a medical student we saw coronary disease only in men who were in their sixties and seventies. We did not see it in young men. But now it is not rare to see a young man in his twenties with coronary thrombosis. In the thirties it is not unusual, and in the forties it is common. The prevalence of circulatory disease among young men of draft age was one of the most shocking revelations of World War II. The manpower loss to the military services due to cardiovascular disease was unbelievable. There were 7 per cent rejections, or 4,000,000 rejectees during the war due to some cardiovascular defect. From July 1950 to July 1951, of all the registrants for military service, 16 per cent were rejected because of cardiovascular disease. From 1942 to 1945, 80,000 men were discharged from service because of cardiovascular disability.

How much of this frightening record was due to compulsive smoking of young men in their late teens and early twenties? How many of our World War II and Korean War veterans will turn up sooner or later at veterans' hospitals as heart and lung-cancer patients?

I am convinced that hundreds of thousands of non-smokers were inducted into the cigarette habit by the generous cigarette makers who patriotically proclaimed on the air their free gifts of millions of cigarettes to our armed forces. I am not alone, apparently, in my apprehensions. Dr. Horace Joules, Director of the famous Middlesex Hospital in London, writes: "Young conscripts tend to smoke excessively at an early age. I wonder how many will die a very painful death before the age of sixty!"

That smoking because of its nicotinic action constricts the blood vessels, increases the heart rate, raises the blood pressure has long been known. That it is a poison, and a killing poison, is not subject to question. Standard textbooks have more and more to say of its malign effects on the cardiovascular system.

Allen, Barker, and Hines in their textbook on "Peripheral Vascular Disease," advise complete abstinence from tobacco in arteriosclerosis. Most leading cardiologists advise against tobacco in patients with angina pectoris, and in coronary thrombosis. Many say that in the control and treatment of *any type* of heart disease, smoking should be absolutely forbidden.

Authorities such as Dr. George E. Burch, of the Tulane University Medical School and of the Charity Hospital in New Orleans, would prohibit smoking in all cases of coronary thrombosis and coronary occlusion.

Of the conditions either caused or aggravated by smoking, one of the most serious is coronary thrombosis—formation of a blood clot in the arteries approaching the heart. Because smoking can cause paroxysms of the arteries of the heart, clotting of the blood in these arteries is favored and nutrition of the heart is impaired.

Dr. John E. Sutton, at a recent panel meeting of New York physicians, offered himself as an example of other ill effects of nicotine. For years he had smoked three or four cigarettes with his morning coffee. One morning he observed that his left arm seemed to be asleep. He believed this had been caused by resting on it during the night. But the numbness failed to disappear. He told a medical conference recently: "I could not shave. I could not dress. I could not tie my necktie. When I regained the use of my hand, I said to my wife that I was going to try an experiment and that it may prove what was wrong with me.

"I had been smoking cigarettes for thirty years. So I picked out one of my favorite cigarettes and began inhaling it, as I usually did. The tip of my thumb and all of my fingers began to tingle. They became dead and white and that tingling and dead feeling went up to my elbow and I was right back where I started from, with a perfectly paralyzed hand and arm. I was admitted to the hospital and had a course of anticoagulants administered. Gradually improvement occurred."

Dr. Sutton never smoked again.

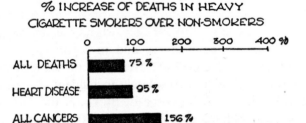

% INCREASE OF DEATHS IN HEAVY
CIGARETTE SMOKERS OVER NON-SMOKERS

Heavy smoking nearly doubles the death rate from heart disease.

The extent of dangers to the vascular system has been depicted vividly by Dr. Grace Roth, of Mayo Clinic, who experimented on what she described as "500 normal people."

Dr. Roth first took the blood pressure, heartbeat, and skin temperatures of the subject, obtained an electrocardiogram, and then gave him corn silk to smoke. Nothing happened. She then invited him to smoke a cigarette of his favorite brand. After the smoke, she examined the patient.

She found that the skin temperatures of the fingertips and toes had dropped from two to six degrees. The pulse rate increased as many as eight beats a minute. Blood pressure increased as much as fifteen millimeters. There were detrimental changes in the electrocardiogram.

The change in skin temperature is especially important: it indicates that the blood vessels in the extremities have contracted. This condition occurs constantly in Buerger's disease, and when it is stimulated further by smoking, the blood circulation is so desperately affected that amputation of a limb is likely.

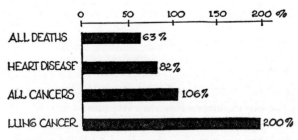

% INCREASE OF DEATHS IN ALL CIGARETTE
SMOKERS (HEAVY & LIGHT) OVER NON-SMOKERS

ALL DEATHS — 63%
HEART DISEASE — 82%
ALL CANCERS — 106%
LUNG CANCER — 200%

"The use of tobacco may mean the difference between life and death for persons with diseases of the circulation."

To all this has now been added the statistical confirmation that indicates the deadly degree to which the nicotine in tobacco has become the weapon for Killer No. 1—heart disease—just as the carcinogenic tars in tobacco smoke have become the active agents of Killer No. 2—cancer.

In the report made by the American Cancer Society it is shown that the chances of one's dying of a coronary attack are increased by 95 per cent by heavy cigarette smoking; the chances of dying from cancer are increased by 156 per cent.

9

THE KING—AND YOU

FOR MORE THAN TWO YEARS, FROM OCTOBER 1949 TO FEBRUARY 1952, the world watched and waited while intermittent bulletins issued by the physicians of His Majesty, King George VI, revealed the increasingly critical illness of England's King.

The official announcements were brief. The first bulletin mentioned a "circulatory-arterial ailment." Subsequent bulletins, in the spring and summer of 1950, spoke of the King's difficulty in walking and of operations designed to restore blood circulation in his legs. Later came announcements of a radiological examination and a lung resection.

Two terms were never used, namely, Buerger's disease and lung carcinoma.

But to specialists these symptoms were all too familiar. King George had been struck down by both acute vascular disease and by the maturing crisis of lung cancer. Cigarettes play a deadly role in both diseases.

The King suffered from Buerger's disease—*thromboangiitis obliterans*. The disease is marked by a spasm of the arteries in the extremities, plus an obliteration or occlusion—a plugging of these arteries. As the circulation in the extremities is cut off, the fingers and toes first turn white and may become gangrenous, necessitating their amputation.

Some of the surgery performed on the King was an attempt to control the spread of this condition. It was relatively beneficial.

Frequently the King had been advised, as are all such patients, to stop smoking. But he could not be persuaded to give up his cigarettes.

Terrible is the grip that smoking addiction may fasten on some of its victims. Recently I advised a patient with Buerger's disease to give up smoking immediately and warned him of the possibility of amputation. "Then you'll have to amputate," he said, "because I am sure I can't stop." I am equally sure that one day I shall amputate.

Nor is mine a rare experience. A well-known physician has remarked: "I marvel how intelligent individuals calmly go about killing themselves." He, too, had thromboangiitis patients who, despite repeated warnings to stop smoking, preferred to lose their legs rather than give up the cigarette habit.

Yet time and again it has been proved that the cessation of smoking results in arresting the disease, and that in early cases giving up cigarettes alone is followed by the complete disappearance of all symptoms.

All smokers eventually develop a cough. A cough is also one of the first symptoms of lung cancer. Unfortunately, too many smokers take their cough too lightly. Often the cough appears to be confined to the throat, and the smoker, red-faced in a coughing siege, merely blames it all on "smokers' throat." Because it is in his throat, he doesn't worry about his lungs.

Cancer of the larynx has increased approximately as rapidly as lung cancer in the past twenty years. The death rate of cancer of the larynx has not increased so sharply simply because the larynx is easier for the doctor to observe and to operate on than the lung.

In lung cancer, the doctor must rely largely on symptoms. The first of these is the cough, but since most smokers aren't disturbed by their cough they don't see their doctors about it. Eventually the cough changes in its sound, becoming more of a chest cough than a throat cough.

Soon afterward the smoker finds himself wheezing with increasing heaviness. His sputum changes in appearance, grows more solid in substance, and may even contain blood. Chances are that the sputum contains cancer cells, and if this is discovered in time the smoker has an opportunity for effective surgery.

As the symptoms progress, the smoker gradually becomes increasingly aware of his chest. There is no pain, but a slight discomfort. It is somewhat like having a nail in your shoe: the preliminary annoyance is slight, but gradually increases. Ordinarily, you don't think of your chest or the process of breathing

COMPARATIVE INCIDENCE OF RECORDED SYMPTOMS

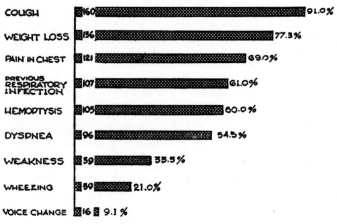

Smokers! Watch for these symptoms.

any more than you watch your feet when you walk. A cancer growth will make itself known.

Months pass. You begin to lose your appetite, lose weight, the chest pain increases, you frequently catch cold, you cough up more blood, and you have difficulty in breathing.

At this point you will probably decide that it might be a good idea to see your doctor. And by this time, if you are a heavy smoker, you will probably have several cancer growths in your lung and in surrounding tissue.

Knowing you have smoked excessively for years, your doctor will strongly suspect what's wrong with you—and he'll be right. But he will want to be sure. He will take X rays of your chest. There is a chance, however, that your cancer is in a part of your lung which does not show clearly in X ray.

The doctor may then try a bronchoscopic examination. This permits him to insert an instrument down your throat through which he will be able to look around the central portions of your lung and make a close study of your tumor, if it is nearby. Other

CARCINOMA OF THE LUNG

TOTAL

OPERABLE 60%

RESECTABLE 36%

SURVIVED RESECTION 26%

FIVE YEAR CURE 8%

No smoker can seek medical advice soon enough if he wishes to live.

equipment on the instrument enables the doctor to nip off a piece of the tumor for microscopic study.

But may be that won't work either. Maybe your cancer is completely inaccessible to any of the present methods of observation. And chances are one to five that this will be the case. Your doctor will have to open you up, or he will refer you to another surgeon who specializes in this delicate operation.

By the time you stretch out on the operating table, you probably will have spent from eight months to two years letting the symptoms of lung cancer develop. Nobody knows how long the cancer has been at work inside you. By waiting, you have lessened your chance of survival.

Let me give you some statistics that I compiled during a relatively brief period in my surgical practice:

Of 1,457 cases of lung cancer brought to me and my colleagues, 668 were considered to be too far gone to warrant even an exploratory operation. Sixty-nine of the 789 who were operable refused surgery; we operated on 723. On getting a close look at them, we found that we could do absolutely nothing for 254 of them.

Survival Rate in Primary Pulmonary Malignancy After Resection

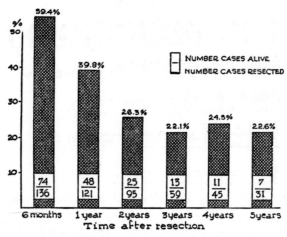

If you are a smoker, do something about it now.

For the remaining 469 there was a chance. Either they were in good enough health otherwise or the cancer had not got out of hand; we decided it was advisable to remove the afflicted lung and, when possible, as many of the metastases (second growths) as we could.

Of these, 89 died in the hospital; 380 were discharged and sent home.

Of our 1,457 patients we were able to help 380. Because the cancers were far advanced in three fourths of the patients from whom we removed the lung, we knew that, of the 380, less than half would be alive at the end of a year. Only 15 per cent (thirty-five) would be alive at the end of five years.

Yet if all of the 1,457 cases had sought the advice of their doctors earlier, in fact as little as six months earlier, chances are we could have cured most of them and prolonged the lives of the rest.

It's not a pretty picture. Nor is it meant to be. FEAR OF CANCER SAVES LIVES was a headline in the Science Newsletter. "A wholesome fear of cancer is a legitimate weapon of no mean power in the fight against cancer," wrote the late Dr. James Ewing, the greatest cancer authority of his day.

That fear was not enough to save King George VI. It may be enough to save you, if you are a smoker and do something about it.

10

MORE COUNTS IN THE INDICTMENT

As significant as the findings which confirm statistically the previous studies of the relationship of smoking to death
from heart and arterial diseases is the conclusion reached in the
American Cancer Society's Hammond-Horn report that

"Cigarette smoking is associated with an increase in
the death rate from most of the common sites of cancer
in men."

Such a conclusion must make for renewed interest in the question: How about smoking and stomach cancer, which lung cancer
has just passed as the leading cause of cancer death in men? Certainly the question must now be fully investigated.

Although the respiratory tree is obviously an area in the body
that is irritated by the tars and resins of tobacco, many medical
men point to the fact that these resins and tars are absorbed in
the saliva and swallowed, and thus are commonly accepted as a
cause for precancerous conditions in the stomach. Tobacco produces an irritation of the gastric mucous membrane, causing a
continuous outpouring of hydrochloric acid which eventually,
under certain circumstances, can cause congestion of the membrane and an ulcer. Often such ulcers become malignant.

The reason why the role of the use of tobacco in the production
of cancer of the stomach is not so generally recognized, it has
been said, is because there are many other factors and causes of

ulcer of the gastrointestinal tract, all of which can be followed by cancer.

The burden that cigarette smoking imposes upon the gastro-intestinal tract and the respiratory system is incontestable. My own experience would indicate that most so-called stomach ulcers are actually ulcers of the first portion of the intestinal tract beyond the outlet of the stomach, which is called the duodenum. But regardless of whether the ulcer is in the stomach or in the duodenum, I have yet to see a patient get well if he continues to smoke. I flatly refuse to treat ulcer patients who do not agree to discontinue smoking.

"The importance of smoking as an irritating factor," Dr. Sara M. Jordan of the Lahey Clinic, in Boston, has written, "is thoroughly recognized by the modern experienced technician; in the author's experience it ranks with fatigue and tension as the most frequent cause of ulcer recurrence, and therefore it [smoking] is completely banned and permanently so."

Ehrenfeld and Sturtevant show that after the smoking of only two cigarettes there is a marked rise in gastric acidity that lasts for more than an hour. Such an authority as Sir Berkeley Moynihan has written: "Among the most harmful of habits for all these [ulcer] patients is smoking," and here Dr. Burrill Crohn, of Mount Sinai Hospital, New York, has called attention to the fact that it often lights up an inactive ulcer.

The throat, which each tobacco company swears is safer in its hucksters' care than in the care of a physician, is irritated by tobacco smoke of any kind.

Dr. Greydon Boyd, of New York University, reported to a recent medical symposium:

"Of eighteen otolaryngologists (ear, nose, and throat specialists) interviewed, 100 per cent believed tobacco to be irritating to the nose and throat."

It is now indisputable that excessive smoking injures the nervous system, is detrimental to digestion, makes for active ulcers as stated earlier in this chapter, encourages blood clot by narrowing the blood vessels, and sometimes causes blindness, as in nicotine amblyopia. The literature is increasing with other symptoms of excessive smoking. Bohan and Berry studied eighty patients who suffered from dizziness, feelings of uncertainty and apprehensiveness, and the "blind staggers"—all symptoms of low blood-sugar levels or hypoglycemia. Nearly half of these patients smoked excessively. Of this half, thirty-six were persuaded to stop smoking; they were free of their hypoglycemia symptoms within a month. One of them had smoked two or three packages of cigarettes daily for forty years. Within a month after stopping smoking all his apprehensions disappeared.

Cigarettes, it would appear from recent literature, cause serious disturbance of many normal bodily functions. Smoke from one or two cigarettes releases into the blood stream a stream of pituitary gland hormones sufficient to constrict the heart of a dog and perhaps of a man. Dr. J. I. Burns, of Oxford University, found that the amount of smoke released by a cigarette or two inhibited the secretion of urine caused by drinking water. But in this brief volume I can treat only of a few counts in the total indictment.

Until recently the association of cigarette smoking to disease has been that of heavy smoking, excessive smoking, persistent smoking over long periods of time.

The Hammond-Horn conclusion, that "even light cigarette smoking is associated with increasing death rates," greatly advanced the indictment against cigarettes. Present figures show that death rates were appreciably higher among men who smoked regularly less than half a pack of cigarettes a day than among men who never smoked.

But it is to be expected that the cigarette makers will go on asking their trick question: "If millions of smokers consume billions of cigarettes, why don't more smokers die of cancer?"

The quick answer might be: "More will—don't worry."

But let's look at the question further: The mounting mortality figures, shocking as they are, do not reveal the full dimensions of the problem. One must take into consideration the morbidity factor in lung cancer.

From a single cell run amok can grow the cancer that will kill you; a vast colony of wild cells may be seen on a pinpoint. Our present diagnostic methods are wholly inadequate to discover cancer at its earliest stages. How many smokers have already acquired the seed of this malignant disease can only be vaguely estimated.

In 1953, according to industry estimate, 3,600 cigarettes per person of smoking age were consumed in this country, a greater per capita consumption than anywhere else in the world. We cannot tell, until they appear at detection clinics, the thousands of determined smokers that would then show the definite symptoms of lung carcinoma.

Except for hospitalized patients, therefore, it is impossible to make any estimate of morbidity in bronchogenic carcinoma. So our positive knowledge must rest on the mortality figures that have now assumed an epidemic character.

An attempted projection recently shown to me—an educated guess at best—indicated a possible total of 200,000 smokers with bronchogenic cancer at the present time in this country.

It could be that—or twice that many.

11

OTHER CAUSES OF LUNG CANCER

NOT EVERY SMOKER WHO DIES AN UNTIMELY DEATH DIES FROM lung cancer. Tobacco smoke is not the only cancer-producing factor that can be inhaled in the lungs with fatal effect. Not every victim of lung cancer was necessarily a smoker.

Dr. Richard Doll, the British investigator, has estimated that about one in five of the lung-cancer deaths in England in 1950 of persons aged twenty-five to seventy-four years was attributable to causes other than smoking; that would leave about 80 per cent which may be considered as caused by smoking. As we have noted earlier, Wynder and Graham reported that, out of 605 cases they had examined, only eight had been non-smokers.

The eagerness of cigarette apologists to accept as completely established the effects on the human body of carcinogens in city smoke contrasts strangely with their refusal to accept the authoritative findings on tobacco as a cancer-producing agent. Yet in all these instances the conclusions rest on empirical evidence and on animal experimentation solely.

There are virtually hundreds of known carcinogens, and it may well be that air pollution is a contributing factor to the incidence of lung disease. It does not explain, however, as the latest American Cancer Society report points out, the observed association between smoking habits and death rates from cancer in rural as well as in urban areas.

In Germany workers in uranium mines were found to show a

disproportionate incidence of lung cancer. German scientists knew that radium could cause cancer and it was soon discovered that uranium, like radium, emitted carcinogenic rays. Preventive steps were taken to protect the workers.

We know that soot and fumes from coal tars contain carcinogens, but during the past twenty years coal consumption in the United States has declined while the mortality from lung cancer has risen. Petroleum consumption, on the other hand, has increased during this period. The sale of fuel oil has risen 350 per cent, and the number of motor vehicles has increased 300 per cent. The exhaust from automobile engines contains a recognized carcinogen, benzpyrene. Other carcinogens have been found in the dust of asphalt roads. Nevertheless, these factors in the environment of modern urban populations thus far have proved insignificant with respect to the incidence of lung cancer.

Why, then, the higher city incidence of lung cancer? Doll and Hill thought various home-heating systems might be involved. But interviews with more than a thousand lung-cancer patients and an equal number of people without the disease failed to turn up appreciable differences among the carcinogenic dangers of heating systems. For a while it was believed by some British scientists that living in the vicinity of a gasworks was a cancer risk. Doll and Hill investigated this, too. They found only a 2 per cent higher case rate among people who lived near gasworks: in this type of survey, the percentage was not considered too significant.

Could lung cancer be an occupational disease? Wynder and Graham studied the possibility, and it appeared, at first, to be likely.

Then these scientists worked up statistics on some 200 patients at the Barnes Hospital Chest Service in St. Louis who were either suspected or known to have been exposed to irritating dusts or fumes on their jobs. About half of them had lung cancer.

The highest incidence seemed to occur among painters: they comprised 5.5 per cent of the lung-cancer group. Also high on the cancer list were hot-metal workers, cold-metal workers, automobile mechanics, carpenters, oilfield workers, miners, electricians, and railroad workers.

In the same St. Louis hospital Wynder and Graham conducted a parallel check on men who presumably had not been exposed to carcinogens on the job. About half had cancer. In this group the highest occupation incidence was among farmers. Clerks, salesmen, executives, accountants, and bartenders were also frequent victims.

The findings were stimulating, but when fully evaluated they did not prove conclusive. Wynder and Graham reported:

"While there are several suggestive relationships, there is no decisive statistical evidence that any of the occupations studied occurs with greater frequency among the cancer patients than among the other chest-disease patients of the Barnes Hospital."

Other groups had come to similarly inconclusive results: an analysis by the Clinical Research Committee of the British Empire Committee in 1944 shows that engineers, mechanics, painters, and decorators are more liable to cancer of the lung than other occupational groups. The Metropolitan Life Insurance Company, studying lung-cancer deaths between 1937 and 1939, lists among the occupations with a higher-than-average death rate engravers, welders, painters, masons, miners, laundry workers, mail carriers, street cleaners, and traveling salesmen.

And as for air pollution, there was this to consider: city men and women inhale the same air. Both sexes should then develop lung cancer at relatively the same frequency. But they do not.

And if air pollution and certain industrial jobs present the greater risks of exposure to carcinogens, then Pittsburgh and St. Louis should have the nation's highest lung-cancer rate. But they do not.

What, then, is the factor that makes the city lung-cancer rate so much higher than the rural incidence?

All surveys show that in practically every lung-cancer case there was one persistent common denominator: tobacco smoking.

Significantly, the preliminary report of the American Cancer

Society showed that essentially the same basic relationships between smoking and cancer were found in the urban and rural groups as were found in the entire population. Such differences as did appear must be considered against the fact that in every age group a larger percentage of men in the rural counties had never smoked and a smaller percentage had a history of regular smoking than was found in urban counties.

At most, the polluted air of cities and the dust and fumes to which certain industrial workers are exposed may be considered *contributing* factors to the high urban incidence of lung cancer.

The basic causative factor is to be found in the carcinogenic properties of tobacco smoke, and of cigarette smoke primarily.

12

FILTERS: A HELP OR A HOAX?

SOMETHING LIKE THE FEAR THAT ONCE COURSED THROUGH great populations at the cry of "The plague!" has tightened the nerves of smokers who are now responding to the double alarm that has been sounded against tobacco abuse. Lung cancer and heart disease, the greatest killers of our time, are now firmly linked to the fantastic increase of cigarette consumption in this country: from 100,000,000,000 units in 1933 to about 400,-000,000,000 in 1954. Massive findings, based on human evidence, associate cancer with the irritant tars in tobacco smoke, and the rising death rate from heart disease with nicotine. These facts, at last, have become public knowledge.

Daily, in every American city and town, doctors are faced with questions like these: Is smoking dangerous to my health? How can I reduce the risk if I continue to smoke? (The $64 question, How can I quit smoking, if I must? is discussed in the next chapter.)

Even the brash youth who throws his quarter on the cigarette counter and says, "Give me a package of cancer sticks!" is likely to have private qualms.

But, for the most part, scared smokers, like the trusting children who followed the Pied Piper of Hamelin, are turning to filter-tip cigarettes, to king-size cigarettes, to king-size filter-tip cigarettes, to "denicotinized" cigarettes, to filter holders, for promised "health protection."

Are these filters a help or a hoax?

Certainly effective filtration, coupled with moderate smoking habits, is to be encouraged—if you must smoke, which I do not recommend. But let's look at the medical record:

Millions who have turned from regular cigarettes to filters made from cotton, crepe paper, asbestos fiber, sulfa-flox, and activated charcoal are smoking twice as much under the illusion that this is "safe" and also in order to get the kick that their nicotine addiction demands. Others smoke the king-size cigarettes to the shortest possible butt, thereby actually increasing their intake of tars and nicotine. Smoked "to the last cool puff," as the advertisements put it, king-size cigarettes make for king-size cancer.

As for the filter holders, the filters are rarely changed often enough to provide significant protection.

Ironically, the perfect filter was discovered—and discarded.

"Our experiments with the new filter (micronite) were fantastic," one of the leading cigarette makers has proclaimed in his advertising. "The material turned out to be so perfect that it filtered out the smoke as well as the tobacco irritants. Nothing came through it but warm air." The filter was quickly "loosened."

That the filters currently available are a hoax rather than a help is evident from independent laboratory findings.

The chemical laboratory of the American Medical Association has investigated the claims of paper, asbestos, and cotton filters, and of the so-called denicotinized cigarettes. It found that very little of the total nicotine in the smoked portion of the cigarette was removed by the cigarette filters that were tested. In fact, the nicotine content of the mainstream smoke of one of the filter-tip brands proved to be exceptionally high—higher than that of "regular" cigarettes. Cigarette tobaccos vary widely in nicotine content.

The term "denicotinized," the laboratory stressed, was a misnomer. To the unitiated "denicotinized" would denote tobacco that is nicotine-free. None of the tobaccos examined were really nicotine-free; there are, in fact, no nicotine-free cigarettes.

The substantial question, however, is whether or not filter-tip or "denicotinized" cigarettes reduce the hazards of smoking.

Dr. Grace M. Roth and her associates at the Mayo Clinic studied the effects of cigarette smoking on the circulatory system. They found that standard American cigarettes contained about 2.5 per cent of nicotine, averaging well over twice as much as West Indian brands, which usually contain less than 1 per cent. Oriental cigarettes were found to contain from 1.25 to 1.5 per cent of nicotine. So-called "denicotinized" cigarettes actually contained more nicotine than some of the West Indian varieties, and only a little less than the ordinary Oriental brands.

When samples of all these cigarettes were smoked, the effects were found to relate directly to the amount of nicotine they contained.

In filters, as the *Journal of the American Medical Association* has editorially declared, "the amount of nicotine and tars that reaches the smoker's oral cavity is the one factor of fundamental importance."

In this respect it's the cigarette huckster, not the scientist, who is likely to control the industry's claims. If so, what the American smoker may confidently expect is an advertising barrage for ever-new miracle filters—filters that will not only filter out the nicotine in tobacco smoke but even the carcinogens which the cigarette industry claims aren't there! New calculations will be contrived to bolster claims for allegedly low percentages of nicotine. Different bases will be chosen for these calculations in order to give different results from the same analytical data. Much of this will be true—technically.

So we shall see the force of Blake's words:

> The truth that's told with bad intent
> Beats all the lies you can invent.

13

YOU *CAN* STOP SMOKING

EVERY TOBACCO USER, WHETHER HE SMOKES STANDARD CIGA-rettes, filter cigarettes, "denicotinized" cigarettes, pipes, or cigars, whether he snuffs tobacco or chews tobacco, is a candidate for cancer. And he will remain a candidate, as long as he uses tobacco in any form.

As stated at the beginning of this book, the amount of tars and other possibly carcinogenic substances you have absorbed daily from tobacco, and the number of years you have irritated the delicate lung tissues by continuous smoking, determine your chances of developing cancer. Heavy smokers often die from heart disease before cancer has reached its inevitable climax. But this does not change the picture; the more you smoke the greater your hazard is a fact now confirmed in the figures presented by the American Cancer Society.

The mature smoker is becoming aware of the awesome risks he is taking. More and more the cry is arising in the medical office, "Doctor, I want to stop smoking, but I can't."

To most patients who say this I have only one answer: "Of course you can! Don't be like the elephant who imagined himself tethered because his keeper had twisted a piece of grass around his leg."

How baseless is the fear that the habit is unbreakable should be quickly apparent from the answer to this question: What would happen if you were stranded without cigarettes on a desert island?

Nothing, of course, except that after a few days of mild craving your digestion would improve, your smoker's throat would clear up, your smoker's cough would disappear, your sight would become clearer, and your "heartburn" would cease. And as your health improved you would forget about cigarettes.

True, saturation with nicotine can turn habit into addiction. The habit-forming drug nicotine was isolated from tobacco in 1822. For more than 100 years its effects have been investigated and studied. Like the opiates, nicotine causes definite physiological changes. The body becomes dependent upon a daily dose of nicotine and tends to want larger and larger doses. This, as repeated demonstrations have proved, is true whether the nicotine has been introduced into the system by smoking or by intravenous injection. Dr. Lennox Johnston, the British investigator and a one-time chain smoker himself, has written in the London *Lancet*: "Addiction to tobacco, like addiction to opium, is a specific disease—an intermittent intoxication."

Whatever the degree of addiction that compulsive cigarette smoking imposes upon its victims, this much is clear: Self-medication is dangerous. If your system needs to be "denicotinized," better place yourself under your doctor's care. Don't rinse your mouth with dangerous chemicals.

The anti-smoking pills, growing in number and variety, coat your mouth and throat with a film that seemingly gives a bad taste to the cigarette smoke. Actually, it is the film you taste.

The old stable-grown remedy, I am told, was much more effective: it was to place a bit of hair from an equine's tail in your cigarette butt, light up, and puff. The first few puffs usually were enough to cure the most hardened smoker. It was an early example of conditioned reflex therapy.

There are as many systems of giving up smoking as there are ways to stop the hiccups.

Here is my own ten-point program:

1. *Stop smoking abruptly, completely, and permanently*

While it is true that some heavy smokers have successfully reduced their consumption of tobacco and then either stabilized their smoking on a moderate level or stopped entirely, "tapering off" is not the method of choice. In the first place, it usually involves greater and more prolonged physiological and psychological discomfort than quitting abruptly and completely. In the second place, the usual relapse into excessive smoking occasions feelings of frustration, humiliation, and guilt.

2. *Know why you smoked*

No habit, including the smoking habit, ever seizes upon its victims. You have acquired the smoking habit, and you continue it for reasons which rarely withstand objective examination. Dr. Gelolo McHugh, Professor of Psychology at Duke University, found that his college students started smoking because they wanted to appear more grown up, to relieve a sense of inadequacy, to attain proper status in a group, to become what they regarded as men and women of the world.

But 70 per cent of these students soon became heavy smokers. They continued to smoke excessively despite their conviction that it was not good for them. Thus a habit learned to satisfy a psychological need became a need in itself—a physiological or pharmacological need.

Ask yourself whether the reasons you give yourself for smoking are good ones. Does smoking really quiet your nerves? Does it relieve fatigue? Is it necessary to your social ease? If you convince yourself, as you should, that the answer must be "No!" your resolution to quit will thereby be strengthened.

3. *Build up your resolution*

If your reasons for smoking were bad, your reasons for quitting the habit are correspondingly good. This or any similar text dealing with the relationship of excessive smoking to disease should provide a multitude of such reasons. I myself have never smoked. But if I had, I cannot imagine myself continuing the habit after my first look at a cancerous lung.

It is to be noted that practically all the scientists who have studied the relationship of smoking to cancer and other diseases have either abandoned the habit, if they were smokers, or adopted what they considered less harmful forms of smoking.

Lennox Johnston writes: "In order to stop, it is necessary to do much more than merely decide. There must be a build-up of resolution sufficient to withstand indefinitely all urges to smoke. As in war, the more overwhelming the preparatory build-up of strength, the easier and more certain the victory."

4. *Burn your bridges to the habit*

Throw away all your smoking paraphernalia: cigarettes, cigars, cigarette holders, pipes, even ash trays and cigarette containers. Tell your friends that you have stopped smoking on the advice of your physician and let them assume anything they choose; at least they'll probably stop offering you cigarettes.

When Gloria Swanson stopped smoking, I am told, she made substantial bets with friends that she wouldn't resume the habit, thereby strengthening her resolution by fear of financial loss.

5. *Time your break*

Illness, especially a cold in the head, seems to lessen the smoker's appetite for tobacco. If the illness is severe enough to keep you at home or in hospital, your opportunity to break the habit is that much better.

The same is true if you can avoid the social and psychological pressure of smokers, because a smoking environment acts both to spread and maintain the habit. You may not be able to afford an extended business trip, a sea voyage, or a wilderness vacation with non-smoking friends to help you break the smoking habit, but eschew as much as possible the companionship of heavy smokers until you are rid of your addiction.

6. *Disregard the brief withdrawal symptoms*

The first day and a half after you have stopped smoking is the crucial period. Deny yourself tobacco that long and you've won half the battle. The pharmacological craving reaches its peak toward the end of the first twenty-four or thirty-six hours. After that it declines sharply and steadily. Remember that no matter how you feel, your withdrawal symptoms are actually signs of recovery from the disease of tobacco addiction. De-toxification is proceeding; that brings an improvement in mental and physical tone which is soon manifest. You will continue to experience intermittent and progressively less acute cravings for tobacco for some weeks or even months. The more contemptuously you treat this craving the less it will bother you.

7. *Adopt substitute habits*

To some extent you can trick the body's craving for tobacco by giving it something else—almost anything except tobacco. When you feel an impulse to smoke, take a drink of water instead. Or reach for a hard candy, an apple, a handful of raisins.

Many have pointed out that there are better ways of relieving tension than by drugging the forebrain with tobacco. The narcotizing effect of nicotine lowers the activity of the forebrain, removes inhibition, and seemingly results in relaxation.

Fresh air, a good walk, agreeable companionship could also relax, without harming the brain and bringing undesirable after-effects. Nicotine is not a therapeutic agent for any purpose; it is a poison, and a killing poison. A lukewarm bath before retiring will often be sufficient to relieve tension.

8. *Psychologize yourself*

After the pharmacological craving for nicotine subsides, as it does within thirty-six hours after you have stopped smoking, you will have to deal with involuntary psychological urges to smoke. These may persist for many months.

Some ex-smokers have reported that they were able to surmount this ordeal by converting it into a kind of intellectual game, involving the progressive exposure of the self-deception that characterizes the smoking habit.

For example, a writer who smokes at his desk persuades himself that he needs a cigarette in order to aid his concentration.

He doesn't. What actually happens is that the cigarette depresses his faculties and blurs his perception, so that he writes less well than if he hadn't smoked.

By realizing this, he could, if he would, rout the psychological tempter.

9. *Count your blessings, and proclaim them*

Almost every ex-smoker testifies that he never realized how much smoking was hurting him until he stopped. Within a few weeks you experience an astonishing accession of high spirits, energy and appetite, and a simultaneous recession of coughing, sniffling, and chest pains due to smoking. Keep careful note of these benefits and call them to the attention of your friends. Point out, too, how much money and time you have saved. Thereby your resolution never to smoke again will be hardened and consolidated.

10. *Help others to free themselves*

Tobacco addiction has been called a communicable disease—in a sense that "the desire to smoke originates from the advocacy of smoking by smokers, much of it unconscious." However, if this addiction is communicable, so is the improved health and self-discipline of the ex-smoker. He can tell others his realization of how much harm smoking once did him and how much better he feels now. By doing this he will strengthen his own determination never to smoke again, not to mention the service he may thus render to others.

It was not too long ago when doctors as a class were among the most avid customers of the cigarette industry. Today, apparently, they are helping, by their own example, to alert their patients to the deadly risks of overindulgence.

It is notable that a survey conducted by Dr. Leonid S. Snegireff of the Harvard School of Public Health, assisted by Miss Olive M. Lombard, thus far has shown that more than 32 per cent of the members of the Massachusetts Medical Society do not now use tobacco; 20 per cent report they use less tobacco than they did five years ago. As significant is the fact that 55.5 per cent of the smokers said they had accepted the idea that smoking accounts for cancer of the lung.

It could be that the present rush of lovely ladies to abandon cigarettes and take up pipe smoking will lead eventually to an unexpected result. The danger of lip cancer, the after-taste, not to mention the after-smell, of pipe smoking, should make it easy to abandon the smoking habit entirely.

14

HOW SMOKERS CAN MINIMIZE
THEIR HEALTH RISKS

ALTHOUGH A CAUSE-AND-EFFECT RELATIONSHIP BETWEEN excessive smoking and cancer has been established, as well as a contributory relationship between smoking and heart disease, not every smoker is bound to die of lung cancer or become a victim of heart disease.

We know, with respect to cancer, that the risk increases with the amount and duration of smoking. Less smoking may delay the onset of the disease; more smoking will hasten it. The incubation period may be ten, twenty, even thirty years, depending upon the susceptibility or resistance of the individual.

Susceptibility, we know, plays a role in the increasing mortality from lung cancer. While the cigarette industry seeks to befog the issue, one of the Big Five advertises, in screaming headlines, that one third of the smoking public—21,000,000 smokers—is particularly sensitive to nicotine and tars which have a deleterious effect upon the health.

Obviously the greatest possible "health protection" from nicotine and tars in tobacco is not to smoke at all, which is my own emphatic recommendation.

Nevertheless, we are encouraged to smoke in times of stress, in moments of contentment, in flashes of danger, and hours of triumph. The invitation to cancer, and sudden death from other causes, comes not only from the advertisements but in the dramas seen in films, the theater, and television. A gesture made out of restlessness or boredom or anxiety has taken on a palliative inference regardless of the medical facts. The facts are that you can't make smoking safe. You can only reduce the risks, and you can do this only be reducing your daily intake of nicotine and tars, if you are a smoker. Hence:

1. *Smoke little*

Only your doctor who knows your health story can suggest *how* little. What is moderate for one person may be excessive for another. For most people three or four cigarettes a day—though I certainly don't recommend them—are probably permissible until you reach your sixties or seventies.

2. *Don't cheat your health with filters*

You do just that when you smoke twice as many filter or denicotinized cigarettes as regular cigarettes, thus aborting any possible benefits from filtration.

Laboratory experiments have shown that even the best filter and denicotinized cigarettes contain enough nicotine seriously to affect an impaired heart or circulatory system.

Discard your king-size before it is smoked dangerously short. The additional half inch of the king-size cigarette means that it contains a fifth more nicotine and tar than the regular-sized cigarette. Smoked to a short butt, the long cigarette is more dangerous than the short or standard cigarette.

3. *Avoid inhaling*

Too much smoke reaches the lung even if you are not consciously inhaling. As already mentioned, it has been established that cancer growths among inhalers occur mostly in the peripheral regions, among non-inhalers in the central regions of the lung. Deliberately inhaling adds greatly to the amount of carcinogens and other tobacco poisons to which you expose the respiratory tract.

Cigarette advertising can be informative. Do you know how many times a day you inhale if you are an average smoker? "The right answer," says a cigarette advertisement, "is 200 times a day—yes, over 200 times every day your nose and throat are exposed to irritation."

4. *Don't hold smoke in your mouth*

Dr. Grace M. Roth of the Mayo Clinic found that when smoke is held in the mouth for two seconds, 6.6 to 7.7 per cent of the nicotine is absorbed in the respiratory passages. Her conclusion: "The amount of nicotine absorbed from one cigarette is dependent on how long the smoke remains in the mouth, whether the smoke is inhaled or not, and the frequency and depth of inhalation."

5. *If you switch to a pipe, keep it clean and cool*

Prominent cancer investigators, sobered by their own findings, have switched from cigarettes to pipes or cigars, to reduce the risk of lung cancer. Graham and Wynder found that the average age of pipe smokers with cancer was 60.5 years—approximately seven years more than the average in cigarette smokers.

Heat, combined with the carcinogenic properties of tobacco, as has been pointed out in a previous chapter, often causes cancer of the lip, tongue, mouth, or larynx. Surveys both here and abroad have shown that though smokers of pipes and holders develop fewer lung cancers they develop more mouth cancers.

Therefore, don't draw too heavily on your pipe; avoid gripping the pipestem in the same area of the mouth during a long period of heavy smoking; keep bowl and stem meticuously clean and free from the muck and poisonous residue of the tobacco.

Pipe smokers generally consume less tobacco than cigarette smokers. Filter holders have proved more effective in the reduction of nicotine and tars than filter-tip cigarettes.

The best practice for the cigar smoker is to throw away the cigar when it is about one third consumed. It has been argued that since inhaling is very common among cigarette smokers and rare among cigar smokers it is likely that the former absorb considerably more nicotine than the latter.

6. *Catch cancer symptoms early*

Again, whether you are a heavy smoker or a light smoker, you can reduce the cancer risk, but not eliminate it.

If you have been a steady smoker, even if you have stopped smoking, it would be wise to have your chest X-rayed immediately for early detection of possible lung cancer in the curable stage. Thereafter, an X ray every six months for at least three years is strongly advisable.

If you are forty and still smoke, even moderately, you should arrange for X rays at four-month periods.

A New York State survey establishes that the risk of lung cancer in men of thirty is doubled among those who smoke less than five cigarettes a day as against non-smokers. The risk is six times greater among those who smoke up to nineteen a day, and ten times greater among heavier smokers. The risk increases proportionately to the number of years of smoking. Men between fifty and sixty who smoke moderately acquire lung cancer from four to fifteen times more often than non-smokers of the same age. Heavy smokers get it from seven to twenty-nine times more. The range of prevalence varies only because scientists vary in their definitions of heavy smoking and because of individual susceptibility.

Early detection and immediate surgery are our best weapons for reducing the mounting mortality from lung cancer. Lung cancers detected in their first stages can be cured; even relatively advanced growths, identified in time, are curable by surgery. The chances are now four out of five that early cancer can be detected by X ray.

The peace of mind that comes from knowing that your X ray is negative is rewarding enough to justify regular examinations. As long as you continue to smoke, moderation and vigilance are your basic protections.

15

THE RESPONSIBILITY OF THE INDUSTRY

"No other industry has a greater responsibility to the public health than the cigarette industry. And none has failed so dismally to discharge its manifest obligations. It hucksters a product that carries disease and death in its wake. Its mendacious advertising has been condemned by the Federal Trade Commission, exposed by the National Better Business Bureau, ridiculed by responsible advertising publications, and denounced by the American Medical Association, whose publications no longer accept cigarette advertising. Even New York's Madison Avenue, the trade center of the advertising business, hangs its head in shame because of the vicious "health claims" made in the cigarette industry. "Quick tests," "trick tests," "double talk," "medical hocus pocus," "fictitious surveys," "paid testimonials," are some of the charges that cigarette advertisers have hurled at each other on the air—and they're all true.

"The flagrant irresponsibility shown by cigarette makers would be impossible but for the fact that the industry operates virtually in a legal no man's land—without self-regulation as in similar industries, without government regulation of any kind, and without recognition, in federal or state law, of what everybody knows: that tobacco smoke can be a death-dealing agent when introduced persistently into the human body."

This is the uncompromising summary, made by Roy Norr,

author of "Cancer by the Carton" in *Reader's Digest* (December 1952), and editor of a highly informative monthly newsletter on the social and economic aspects of the problem.*

The fact may well be that the cigarette industry has too long allowed itself to be led by the nose by unprincipled agencies. There are leaders in the industry fully aware of the dread responsibility which the latest scientific findings have brought to their door. Whatever they feel obliged to say for public consumption, these leaders would welcome, I am told, some form of legislative action, state or federal, that would bring the processing and sale of their product under the discipline now imposed upon the liquor and drug industries.

Certainly the fiduciary responsibility of tobacco management is enormous. The industry has a sales volume of more than $5,000,000,000. It gives employment directly or indirectly to millions of people. The tax collector takes a bite of more than $2,000,000,000 annually in taxes. Furthermore, at this writing, Uncle Sam dolefully holds in storage more than 800,000,000 pounds of tobacco, the surplus growth of our tobacco farmers.

A leading tobacco trade journal has estimated that by 1984 the population in the United States will be 200,000,000, of which 140,000,000 will then qualify as smokers. "As a greater number, percentagewise, of the younger generation become cigarette smokers, and as the number of female smokers is enlarging more rapidly than the male counterpart, it can well be expected that a minimum of 70 per cent of both males and females will be smoking by 1984," says *Tobacco*.

The cigarette makers must know that this golden future will fade as continuing research makes it impossible for the industry to ignore the link between persistent smoking and the increasing death rate from cancer and heart disease. They must know that they face the Revolt of the Smoker, now being led by the rank and

* NORR NEWSLETTER about Smoking and Health, 11 West 42nd Street, New York City.

file of the medical profession, which, as indicated by the recent Massachusetts survey, is changing its smoking habits faster than any other segment of the population.

The tobacco industry can at least take a leaf from the experience of other industries. The hard liquor industry has had the grace to advertise to its customers not to take that one drink too many. Many proprietary remedies advertise with the injunction: "Avoid excessive use—follow the directions on label."

The grisly success of the American cigarette industry has been achieved by the deliberate preaching of addiction.

Follow the pattern of its atrocious advertising: it began after World War I with the offer of cigarettes as a health-giving agent, mind you.

Remember? Smoke to aid digestion "during, after and between meals"; smoke for a lift because it "picks up, perks up, renews and restores your energy"; smoke for vim and vigor, as athletes, famous champions and other sports winners do; smoke "to comfort your nerves."

Then followed a phase when cigarettes were sold as a cure-all. Merely switching your brand made "coughs due to smoking entirely disappear." You were told to smoke "as often as you please and as freely as you please"; exhorted to smoke all you wanted "without the thought of irritation"; urged to become "a two pack-a-day smoker."

Next came a period of almost embarrassing confession. You were asked solicitously: "Is your smoking associated with a nagging cough? A dragged-out feeling? Do you lose your taste for food?" (All these are recognized danger signals of possible lung cancer.) You are warned, in big black headlines, that "A FILTER ALONE IS NOT ENOUGH." You are urged, "START TODAY TO SMOKE WITH GREATER PEACE OF MIND."

Today, the larger cigarette companies have leaped almost as one into the tainted pool of paid testimonial advertising concentrated on youth. Everybody smokes on television. Youth's favorite movie stars, pin-up girls, baseball heroes, sports champions drool their pleasure through a haze of smoke. Cigarette smoking is made to confer sophistication upon the girls and manliness upon the boys. Entrancing girl posters are shown that link the ideas of charm and beauty with smoking. College publications are full of cigarette advertising, with brand popularity surveys "supervised by college professors." The young songstress—"everybody's sister"—who jingles be happy, go lucky, luckily avoids her own prescription. She doesn't smoke.

Never has the cigarette industry made a more blatant appeal to youth than in its present advertising; it is almost as if it despaired of keeping adult smokers much longer in leash. The late George Washington Hill, President of the American Tobacco Company, who besought the American flapper to "Reach for a Lucky instead of a Sweet," would have shrunk from the charge that he was introducing youth to the smoking habit. "I should be shocked as anyone else," he protested, "if a tobacco company should undertake to appeal to adolescents."

In view of this record, little note need be taken of the industry's attempts to repudiate the findings of leading cancer scientists here and abroad. These findings have established beyond doubt the critical association between smoking and cancer and smoking and heart disease.

Industry apologists go back to 1923, to 1932, to cite outdated medical testimony in some of their statements, ignoring the accumulated human and experimental evidence which thirty years later, twenty years later, has brought many striking reversals of medical opinion.

Those responsible for establishing the deadly hazards to health which smoking abuse has brought can afford to ignore the meretricious press agentry which dismisses their sober conclusions as "loose talk." The now historic studies of Dr. Graham of St. Louis and of Professor Hill of London, not to mention many others, will survive efforts to obscure their significance. As for my own clinical observations and studies over a period of twenty years, I am content to let the record speak for itself.

It has been said that where the Mayor is the baker, the breads are always small. The Tobacco Industry Research Committee at last has revealed its basic program:

"1. Study of the physical and chemical composition of tobacco and accompanying products;

"2. Study of tissue changes in humans and in animals under various conditions;

"3. Study of smoking and other tobacco habits and of the emotional and physical makeup of smokers."

Of course, the critical areas of investigation, as every research scientist knows, have to do with the problem of how to make smoking a less lethal agent in lung cancer incidence and a less deadly killer in heart disease. Yet it is precisely these areas that apparently have been declared out of bounds for the industry's research committee.

Some measure of the cigarette industry's determination to establish the truth about smoking may be found in the funds it has provided for this work. The sum appropriated to the Tobacco Industry Research Committee for the first year was $500,000— this from a $5,500,000,000-a-year business with a fearful responsibility to public health. It is notable that the much smaller British tobacco industry made a first contribution of $700,000 to research, when the British minister of health announced in Parliament that the association between smoking and cancer must be considered as established. And made it to the British Medical Research Council, not to a hand-picked industry committee. Even in tiny Denmark, the leading cigarette manufacturer contributed last year $200,000 for independent research, when the tragic association between cancer and smoking was made evident in the Doll-Hill report.

It is understandable that the cigarette industry should hope to postpone a day of reckoning for the irresponsible advertising and sale of its products. But a tapeworm research into the "physical and chemical composition of tobacco," when an enormous literature already exists on this and similar subjects of its prospective investigation, is not likely to save it. The time is coming, I believe, when the legal responsibility of the tobacco companies to their customers will have to be clarified. "For if it is an offense to produce foods which are harmful to the health of consumers," writes a leading authority on cigarette addiction, "it is an offense to produce smoking products which are too often deadly to those who use them."

If the many human studies, now topped by the massive survey of the American Cancer Society, do not resolve the medical "controversy" over smoking which the immense economic power of the tobacco industry keeps alive, sooner or later the courts must decide the responsibility of the industry on the weight of scientific evidence which is now beyond any reasonable doubt. In this event, "chimney sweeps' cancer" might serve as a significant precedent.

In 1775, Sir Percivall Pott, famous British military surgeon, described cancer of the scrotum as the occupational disease of the unfortunate little chimney sweeps. He wrote in his book, *Chirurgical Observations:*

"The fate of these people seems singularly hard. In their early infancy they are most frequently treated with great brutality, and almost starved with cold and hunger; they are thrust up narrow and sometimes hot chimneys, where they are bruised, burned and almost suffocate; and when they get to puberty become peculiarly liable to a most noisome, painful and fatal disease."

He found that the disease "derives from the lodgment of soot in the rugae of the scrotum." It was called "soot-wart" in the trade, he wrote, and mistakenly treated with mercurials for venereal disease.

Though the chemical discovery of benzpyrene, a virulent carcinogen in coal, came more than one hundred and fifty years later, British courts and other courts throughout the world accepted the cause-and-effect relationship of coal soot to cancer and established that chimney sweeps or their families were entitled to workmen's compensation, if the chimney sweeps contracted the disease.

The law did not wait for "irrefutable" scientific proof; the mineowners sent up no cry that coal soot was maligned; and the coal barons did not dismiss Sir Percivall's clinical findings as merely "loose talk."

It would be preposterous to say that the cigarette industry does not want to remove death-dealing substances from tobacco smoke. But it would be equally preposterous to accept its unblushing insistence that smoking is harmless.

Yet the very first statement announcing the formation of the Tobacco Industry Research Committee contained this declaration: "We believe the products we make are not injurious to health."

Even if it were possible to dismiss the repeated findings here and abroad, so dramatically confirmed by the American Cancer Society's figures, indicating that smoking more than doubles the death rate from cancer and nearly doubles the death rate from coronary disease, there's the incontestable fact that light smoking, not to mention heavy smoking, may have upon many a deleterious effect upon health.

Records kept by the Life Extension Examiners show that smokers complained of cough 300 per cent more often than non-smokers, that they complained of nose and throat disease 167 per cent more often than non-smokers, of palpitation 50 per cent more often, of pain over the heart 73 per cent more often, of heartburn 100 per cent more often, of nervousness 76 per cent more often than non-smokers.

A realistic and cooperative attitude on the part of the cigarettemakers would serve the best interests of the tobacco industry as well as the smoking population. The industry, I believe, would be well advised to support such steps as the following:

First, the production and sale of tobacco products should be studied by Congress with the idea of bringing tobacco within the purview of regulation that now protects consumers of alcoholic beverages and drugs.

Cigarette smoke contains nicotine, a highly poisonous alkaloid, carbon monoxide, acrolein, ammonia, prussic acid and aldehydes grouped under the term "tars," generally recognized as cancer-producing sources. Proper labeling would give the smoker information about the active poisons in tobacco to which he is clearly entitled.

Second, smokers should be warned, in cigarette advertising, against the dangers of tobacco abuse.

The industry is inescapably obligated to recognize the health hazards of a habit-forming product that is sold indiscriminately to teenagers, adolescents and adults alike.

Third, testimonial advertising should be outlawed completely by the cigarette industry.

The Association of National Advertisers has on record a resolution adopted in 1929, declaring: "We view with disapproval the use of the so-called paid testimonials." The resolution was passed during an earlier outbreak of cigarette testimonial advertising. An advertising authority has stated: "As long as people in the mass are what they are the actions of millions of them can be controlled by any reiterated claim."

Smoking addiction is a disease, and testimonial advertising communicates that disease, unfairly and irresponsibly to emulative youth.

Fourth, the industry should take all possible measures to discourage the use of cigarette dispensing machines.

It was not long ago when youth began smoking at eighteen or twenty; today boys and girls of ten or twelve begin this destructive habit, aided by these one-armed addiction pushers which, in effect, abrogate state and local laws against the sale of cigarettes to minors.

Would the measures I have suggested "ruin" the cigarette industry? Hardly. There's little danger that the tobacco industry will run out of customers.

Not as long as there are smokers who will deliberately suffer quadruple amputation, rather than heed the warning to quit smoking—or else.

16

CANCER CAN BE CONQUERED

DESPITE OUR BETTER DIAGNOSIS OF MALIGNANT TUMORS, THE perfection of our surgical techniques and the recent advances in radiation therapy, the *causes* of many cancers remain locked in the mystery of cell growth.

Nevertheless, many cancers *can* be prevented.

In the case of lung cancer, the most dreaded and deadly form of malignant disease, prevention is the key to the problem—the key that has hung almost unused outside the door.

In 1928 the late Dr. James Ewing, famous pathologist and cancerologist, wrote:

"One may hardly hope to eliminate the tobacco habit, but cancer propaganda should emphasize the danger signs that go with it."

That was when the lung cancer mortality rate had barely begun its steep and ominous climb, paralleling the huge increase in the consumption of cigarettes in this country. Today we know, through human studies and animal experimentation, that the key to the control of the present lung cancer epidemic lies in a fundamental change in our smoking habits.

Those who have a vested interest in keeping the truth about smoking and health from the American people have now raised the cry of "Cancerophobia!", as if those who sought to place the facts before the public were scaremongers. Dr. Ewing, in his time, brushed such charges aside. In his classic essay on Cancer Prevention, he stated:

"The cancerophobia which attends all publicity about cancer is of very minor importance. A wholesome fear of cancer is a necessary attribute of all educated men and women, and its excessive indulgence belongs mostly to those who are naturally inclined to cultivate this or other psychoses."

He urged that all possible means of control be adopted in the interest of self-preservation.

Pasteur was credited with saying that when he approached the problem of disease his first thought was, How can it be prevented? not, How can it be cured?

Since Pasteur spoke, preventive medicine has passed from one triumph to another, while curative medicine often struggles vainly against the inertia of established pathological processes.

Last year there were few to challenge the statement of Dr. James Stevens Simmons, Dean of the Harvard University School of Public Health, when he charged that all too often preventive medicine was treated as a stepchild of modern medical practice, with the result that millions of people here and abroad suffered needless deaths and avoidable disease. "A fog of confused thinking," said Dr. Simmons, "has delayed the full development of adequate health protection and the acceptance of the simple truth that an ounce of prevention is really worth a pound of cure."

Emphasizing the role of prevention in bronchogenic carcinoma, Dr. W. C. Hueper, of the National Cancer Institute, who regards tobacco as only a little bit cancer producing, nevertheless has declared:

"Since an effective arrest of the rising tide of deaths from cancer of the lung cannot be achieved by the presently available diagnostic and therapeutic procedures it becomes imperative to apply preventive measures wherever this is feasible, so as to eliminate or reduce contact with known environmental respiratory carcinogens."

No clinical observation has been more amply confirmed over the years than Ewing's dictum in 1928 that cancer of the larynx was caused mainly by the use of tobacco, and that among the most obvious preventable cancers are those affecting the lip, tongue, floor of the mouth and throat.

There are hopeful signs that the new era of cancer prevention now dawning will have true organizational leadership. Dr. E. Cuyler Hammond, Statistical Director of the American Cancer Society, finds that every bit of evidence so far available fits the hypotheses that smoking and lung cancer and smoking and heart disease are matters of cause-and-effect.

Dr. Charles S. Cameron, Medical Director of the American Cancer Society, as a result of the recent ACS report, has urged youth not to take up smoking and advised beginners to stop smoking.

An immense task faces the health community. More than 230,-000 Americans will die of cancer during this year of 1954. The disease will bring unparalleled fear and suffering, and cost the nation billions of dollars. If nothing is done to arrest the present trend, one in five of us is doomed to develop cancer—perhaps you, I, or both of us.

But a new chapter is opening in our attack upon this disease: the almost unlimited possibilities of life-saving presented by *cancer prevention*. To realize these possibilities the preventive program must be broadly organized.

First, comes the educational problem. It should be studied, I believe, by a commission of educators, public health authorities, temperance workers and physicians appointed by the President of the United States.

Next comes the problem of mobilizing the moral forces of the nation. The abandonment or change of a national habit like smoking is not solely a medical problem; it is a task also for the churches and their educational organizations and instruments.

Third, the program should mobilize the service clubs and fraternal organizations of the country, recruiting from their million-fold membership "minute men"—and women—to help carry on the task.

Fourth, must come a study, by some national conference on cancer prevention, of the role played by our mass communication industries in inducing tobacco addiction with its entailed disease hazards. Not all are willing and eager accomplices to the crime of irresponsible advertising shockingly directed against the health and welfare of the American people.

The press very largely has abandoned its earlier censorship of findings that linked smoking with disease; a few national magazines for the first time have opened their columns to articles on this subject; many publications have shown a decent restraint in the claims they will allow in cigarette advertising.

But on television where the broadcasters are the lessees of the people's air, the cigarette huckster can do no wrong. Every false slogan, every dangerous health claim, every dishonest testimonial that has marked cigarette advertising has appeared on the living screen. The network leaders who control our radio channels are not to be regarded as stuffed parakeets in the gilded cage of cigarette advertising; they have the power to put an immediate stop to the vicious misuse of the air. They have banned, in the public interest, the advertising of hard liquor on their facilities; they can do no less with the evil tobacco advertising that draws youth into the web of cigarette addiction.

Since the publication last June of the American Cancer Society's preliminary study, the causal base for cancer prevention has been broadened by new findings reported to the United Nations Conference on Population, in Rome. Dr. Sully Charles Marcel Ledermann of the French National Institute of Demographic Study in Paris declared that excessive use of tobacco and alcohol appeared to multiply each other as cancer factors. Dr. Ledermann reported:

"Tobacco appears to be an etiological factor in tumors of the buccal cavity and of the respiratory system, also skin cancers of the face. On cancers of the lung in particular, our findings are in agreement with those recently published in Great Britain and the United States.

"A special study was undertaken on how 'the alcohol risk alone' with alcoholics but non-smokers combines with the 'tobacco risk alone' with smokers but non-alcoholics, into a complex 'alcohol-tobacco risk' for alcoholic smokers.

"If, on the one hand, a non-drinking smoker has, for instance, five times more chance to have cancer of the buccal cavity than a non-smoker nor drinker, and, if, on the other hand, a non-smoking alcoholic has five times more chance to have a cancer of the buccal cavity than a non-smoker nor drinker, an alcoholic smoker seems to have not five plus five times more chance to have cancer of the buccal cavity than a non-smoker nor drinker but five times five or twenty-five times more chance."

The complementary effects of smoking and alcohol were observed more than one hundred and fifty years ago by the famous American physician, Dr. Benjamin Rush, who declared in 1798 that smoking and chewing provoked drunkenness. The late Dr. Osler wrote fifty years ago: "Many alcoholic patients in whom the attacks seems to be without exciting cause, if questioned closely, are found to be great tobacco smokers, and the cause of that outbreak is really a recurrent poisoning by tobacco. Usually the history is that they smoke, especially the cigarette smokers, incessantly and to excess. This finally makes them nervous. Then they smoke more to quiet their nervousness until finally they seek another narcotic to quiet them. Then they naturally turn to alcohol."

On many fronts research is advancing toward the conquest of cancer. New anti-cancer drugs have been developed, and hormones and radioactive isotopes have been applied to the treatment of malignant disease. To be sure, the anti-cancer drugs are effective mostly against the lymphomas and the sex steroids act only against a few kinds of carcinomas. But many of these agents have distinct palliative value.

Cancer, with the exception of leukemia and most lymphomas (lymph gland cancers), begins as a local disease and if diagnosed before spread to other parts of the body has occurred, it can be cured by complete surgical removal of the cancer, or by destroying it with X-rays or radium.

Even in cases with extensive local spread much can be accomplished at the present time by undergoing radical surgical removal.

Equally remarkable are some of the advances in radiation therapy, many of them by-products of research on atomic energy. We now have drugs which given orally produce measurable clinical improvement in chronic leukemia and Hodgkin's disease. There is much life-saving promise, too, in the current efforts to develop means of early cancer detection on a mass scale. But the solution to the problem of specific anti-cancer therapy must await a better understanding not only of the metabolism of cancer cells but of the mechanism of normal growth as well.

Ultimately the mystery within the mystery which in immense darkness hides the genesis and mechanism of malignant cell growth will yield, as have other mysteries, to mass attack launched from every possible direction by the combined forces of science.

Yet even if the enigma were solved tomorrow, prevention would still remain better than cure.

In lung cancer, the road to prevention is open and brightly lighted by the cumulative findings of a whole generation of cancer researchers. The means of prevention are at hand.

In cancer of the lung, the source of the major death risk has been established: it is the incessant irritation of the lungs, over a considerable period of time, by the carcinogenic factor or factors that lurk in tobacco smoke. Even those who still suspend judgment on the cause-and-effect relationship of smoking to cancer, agree with authorities here and abroad that, as stated by the *British Medical Journal,* "the younger generation will have to decide, each for himself or herself, whether the additional risk of contracting lung carcinoma is worth taking."

It is for you to decide whether you value smoking more than your lungs or your life. You can prevent smoker's cancer by the simple act of stopping smoking if you are a beginner, or you can reduce this deadly hazard by cutting down tobacco consumption to what your doctor may determine is your tolerance level.

"I should be elated," writes a distinguished scientist in a personal communication, "if I could synthesize a drug which would cure as many cases of cancer as the data indicate could be prevented by the discontinuance of smoking. People do not hesitate to give up eating raw cabbage or water snails in areas where they carry internal parasites. Why should we take the risk of causing lung cancer by smoking?"

"Of the six forms of cancer on which the American Cancer Society is now concentrating," the Society announces, "cancer of the lung has shown the most dramatic and challenging increase." Yet cigarette apologists for years have tried to postpone, with their "doubts," the verdict of science on preventable cancer.

Again, the truly devastating question comes from Roy Norr, the first lay writer to sound an effective alarm about smoking and cancer.

He has written:

"We have become a nation of coughers, sneezers, snifflers, spitters—and the greatest consumers of tobacco products in the world. You can spot the dishonest—and honest—doubters of whether smoking has been proved the Great Killer in cancer and heart disease by asking: To whom would they give the benefit of their doubt? To money or to men? To poison or to people?"

Cancer will be conquered. Better still, it will be *prevented,* as we learn to understand its profound and baffling causes. In lung cancer human studies and animal experimentation, in my opinion, already have placed the key of prevention in our hands. It should be used—promptly and widely—with all the energy and resources at our command.

In my capacity as surgeon and teacher largely concerned with cancer and pre-cancerous conditions, too often I am obliged to deal with the techniques of last resort, oppressed by the conviction that the lives of hundreds of men and women could have been saved by *prevention,* through the abandonment or control of a useless, wasteful and dangerous habit; that these men and women never should have been obliged to come to me.

May the day come when the lung cancer surgeon will be a useless appendage to the medical profession.

Perhaps that is why I have written this book.

REFERENCES

A Study of Cigarettes, Cigarette Smoke and Filters. *J.A.M.A.*, July 11, 1953.

A Study of Cigarettes, Cigarette Smoke and Filters. *J.A.M.A.*, July 4, 1953.

Adler, I.: Primary Malignant Growths of the Lungs and Bronchi. New York, Paul B. Hoeber, 1912.

Buerger, Leo: The Circulatory Disturbances of the Extremities. W. B. Saunders Company, 1924.

Campbell, A. M.: The Effect of Excessive Cigarette Smoking on Maternal Health. *American Journal of Obstetrics and Gynecology,* March, 1936.

Carroll, Frank D.: Etiology and Treatment of Tobacco-Alcohol Amblyopia, *American Journal Ophthalmology,* July, 1944.

Consumers Reports: Cigarettes, February, 1953.

Council for the international organizations of medical sciences under the auspices of the World Health Organizations and United Nations Educational, Scientific and Cultural Organizations: Recommendations adopted by the symposium on the endemiology of cancer of the lung. *Cancer Research,* June, 1953.

Doll, R., and Hill, A. B.: A Study of the Aetiology of Carcinoma of the Lung. *British Medical Journal,* December, 1952.

Doll, R., and Hill, A. B.: Smoking and Carcinoma of the Lung. *British Medical Journal,* September, 1950.

Editorial: Smoker's Larynx. *J.A.M.A.*, March 29, 1952.

Editorial: Smoker's Respiratory Syndrome. *J.A.M.A.*, January 23, 1954.

Editorial: Doll-Hill Study. *New Eng-land Journal of Medicine,* September 10, 1953.

Editorial: Smoking and Lung Cancer. *British Medical Journal,* December 13, 1952.

Ehrenfeld, Irving and Mills Sturtevant: The Effect of Smoking Tobacco on Gastric Acidity. *American Journal of the Medical Sciences,* January, 1941.

Essenberg, J. M.: Cigarette Smoke and the Incidence of Primary Neoplasm in the Lung of the Albino Mouse. *Science,* November 21, 1952.

Forkner, Claude E.: The Harmful Effects of Tobacco. *New York Medicine,* May 5, 1954.

Friedell, Morris T.: Effect of Cigarette Smoke on the Peripheral Vascular System. *J.A.M.A.*, July 4, 1953.

Graham, E. A.: Primary Cancer of the Lung with Special Consideration of Its Etiology. Bulletin of the New York Academy of Medicine. Vol. 27, 1951.

Hammond, E. Cuyler: The Place of Tobacco in the Etiology of Lung Cancer. *CA,* March, 1954.

Hammond, E. Cuyler, and Horn, Daniel: Tobacco and Lung Cancer. *CA,* May, 1952.

Hammond, E. Cuyler: Smoking in Relation to Lung Cancer—A Follow-up Study. *Connecticut State Medical Journal,* January, 1954.

Hammond, E. Cuyler, and Horn, Daniel: Relationship of Human Smoking Habits and Death Rates. *Journal of the American Medical Association,* August 7, 1954. Survey of 186,000 cases.

International Cancer Conference: Sao Paulo, Brazil, July, 1954.

Johnston, Lennox: Cure of Tobacco Smoking. London *Lancet,* September 6, 1952.

Korteweg, R.: The Fight against Lung Cancer. *Documenta de Medicina Geographica et Tropica,* June, 1953.

Ledermann, Sully Charles Marcel, at World Population Conference, Rome, August, 1954.

Levin, M. L., Goldstein, H., and Gerhardt, P. R.: Cancer and Tobacco Smoking. *J.A.M.A.,* Vol. 143, 1950.

Lieb, Clarence William: Safer Smoking. Exposition Press, New York, 1954.

Moore, George E., Bissinger, Lester H., and Proehl, Elsa C.: Intraoral Cancer and the Use of Chewing Tobacco. *Journal of the American Geriatrics Society,* July, 1953.

Norr, Roy: NORR NEWSLETTER about Smoking and Health, 11 West 42nd St., N. Y. C.

Ochsner, Alton: Bronchogenic Carcinoma. *Journal of the Kansas Medical Society,* August, 1950.

Ochsner, Alton: Early Recognition of Bronchogenic Carcinoma. *Postgraduate Medicine,* March, 1953.

Ochsner, Alton, DeBakey, Michael, and Dixon, J. Leonard: Primary Cancer of the Lung. *J.A.M.A.,* October 11, 1947.

Ochsner, Alton, DeCamp, Paul T., DeBakey, M. D., and Ray, C. J.: Bronchogenic Carcinoma—Its Frequency, Diagnosis, and Early Treatment. *J.A.M.A.,* March 1, 1952.

Ochsner, Alton, and DeBakey, Michael: Significance of Metastasis in Primary Carcinoma of the Lungs. *Journal of Thoracic Surgery,* April, 1942.

Perlman, H. H., et al.: The Excretion of Nicotine in Breast Milk and Urine from Cigarette Smoking. *J.A.M.A.,* November 28, 1942.

Pott, Percivall: Chirurgical Observations Relative to the Cataract, Polypus of the Nose, the Cancer of the Scrotum, Mortification of Different Kinds of Ruptures and the Mortification of the Toes and Feet. London, 1775.

Roffo, A. H.: Development of a Carcinoma of the Rabbit Under Influence of Tobacco. *Abs. Am. J. Cancer,* 1931.

Roth, Grace M.: Tobacco and the Cardiovascular System. Springfield, Illinois, Charles C Thomas Publishing Co., 1951.

Snegireff, Leonid S., and Lombard, Olive M.: Survey of Smoking Habits of Massachusetts Physicians. *New England Journal of Medicine,* June 17, 1954.

Sontag, L. W., and Wallace, R. F.: Effect of Cigarette Smoking During Pregnancy Upon Fetal Heart Rate. *American Journal of Obstetrics and Gynecology,* 1935.

Waldbott, G. L.: Smoker's Respiratory Syndrome: A Clinical Entity. *J.A.M.A.,* April 18, 1953.

Wynder, E. L., and Graham, E. A.: Tobacco Smoking as a Possible Etiologic Factor in Bronchogenic Carcinoma—A Study of 684 Proved Cases. *J.A.M.A.,* Vol. 143, 1950.

Wynder, E. L., Graham, E. A., and Croninger, A.: The Experimental Production of Cancer with Cigarette Tar. *Cancer Research,* December, 1953.

Wynder and Graham: Etiologic Factor in Bronchiogenic Carcinoma, With Special Reference to Industrial Exposures—Report of 857 Proved Cases. Archives of Industrial Hygiene and Occupational Medicine, September, 1951.

Wynder and Cornfield: Cancer of the Lung in Physicians. *New England Journal of Medicine,* March 22, 1953.

INDEX

Abortion, 28
Addiction to smoking, 41, 58, 75
Adenocarcinoma, 12, 26
Adler, Dr. I., 12
Advertising, 56, 64, 65, 68, 70-71, 72, 75, 79
Age: blood volume change and, 27; lung cancer and, 15, 26
Air pollution, 50, 51, 52
Alcohol, smoking and, 79-80
Alvarez, Dr. Walter C., quoted, 5-6
Amblyopia, 2, 48
American Cancer Society, 1, 4, 82; research report of, 6-8, 12, 13, 19, 30, 35, 39, 46, 48, 50, 52-53, 73, 74
American Journal of Obstetrics and Gynecology, 27
American Medical Association, 6, 30, 55, 68
Amputation, 39, 40, 41
Antibiotic treatment, 10
Anti-cancer drugs, 80
Anti-smoking pills, 58
Arteriosclerosis, 36
Association of National Advertisers, 75
Asthma, Smoker's, 2

Benzpyrene, 23, 51, 73
Biopsy, 9
Bissinger, Dr. Lester L., 33
Blindness, 2, 48
Blood clot, 36, 37, 47
Blood pressure, high, 36, 38-39
Blood volume, changes in, 26-27
Boyd, Dr. Greydon, quoted, 47
British Committee on Cancer and Radiotherapy, 16-17
British Medical Journal, quoted, 5, 81
British Medical Research Council, 72; Doll-Hill survey for, 14-15, 16 (*see also* Doll-Hill report)
Bronchogenic carcinoma, 10, 14, 77; *see also* Lung cancer
Bronchoscopic examination, 43
Buerger's disease, 39, 40, 41
Burch, Dr. George E., 37
Burns, Dr. J. I., 48

Cameron, Dr. Charles S., 78; quoted, 4, 6
Campbell, Dr. A. M., 27
Cancerophobia, 54, 76-77
Carcinogens, 9, 20, 21, 22, 23, 50-51, 52, 53, 57, 73
Cardiac diseases. *See* Heart disease
Cerebral hemorrhage, 2
Chain smokers, 3, 31
Chewing tobacco, 33, 80
"Chimney sweeps' cancer," 73
Chirurgical Observations (Pott), quoted, 73
Churchill, Winston, 32
Cigarette industry, responsibility of, 68-75
Cigarettes: consumption of, 11, 12, 18, 19, 49, 54; dispensed by machines, 75; disturbance of normal bodily functions by, 48; donated to armed forces, 36-37; filtered and "denicotinized," 54-56, 65; ingredients of smoke of, 74-75; lip cancer from, 34; and stomach ulcers, 47; varia-
tion in individual use of, 3, 8, 13, 31; *see also* Cigar smoking and Pipe smoking
Cigar smoking, 30, 31-34, 66
Circulatory diseases, 2, 36, 40
Clinical Research Committee of the British Empire Committee, 52
Coal, carcinogens in, 50, 73
Coronary diseases, 8, 35, 36, 37, 74
Cough, Smoker's, 2, 41, 74
Crohn, Dr. Burrill, 47
Croninger, A., 20

Death rates, 1, 4, 7, 8, 11-12, 15, 35, 36, 46, 48, 52, 54, 69, 74, 78
DeBakey, Dr. M. E., 18, 19
DeCamp, Dr. Paul T., 18
"Denicotinized" cigarettes, 54, 55-56, 65
Digestion, effect of smoking on, 2, 47
Doll, Dr. Richard, 14, 15, 31, 50, 51
Doll-Hill report, 14-15, 16, 25, 30, 72
Druckrey, 22
Duodenal ulcers, 47

Ehrenfeld, Irving, 47
Epidermoid cancer (Smoker's Cancer), 12, 24, 26
Essenberg, Dr. J. N., 21; quoted, 28
Ewing, Dr. James, quoted, 45, 76, 77

Fetal heartbeat, 28
Filters, 32-33, 54-56, 65, 66
Forkner, Dr. Claude E., quoted, 16
Friedell, Dr. Morris, 26, 27
Frigidity, 28

Gastrointestinal ulcers, 46-47
George VI, King of England, 40-41, 45
Gerhardt, Dr. P. R., 31
Goldstein, Dr. H., 31
Graham, Professor Evarts A., 13, 20, 25, 31, 50, 51, 52, 66, 71
Grant, Ulysses S., 30-31
Greenberg, 33

Habit of smoking: breaking of, 57-63; substitute habits for, 61
Haggard, 33
Hammond, Dr. E. Cuyler, 6, 30, 78; quoted, 8
Hammond-Horn report, 6-8, 12, 13, 19, 30, 35, 39, 46, 48, 50, 52-53, 73, 74
Heartbeat, fetal, 28
Heart disease, 2, 5, 6, 35-39, 54, 57
Heller, Dr. J. R., quoted, 16
High blood pressure, 36, 38-39
Hill, Professor A. Bradford, 14, 15, 25, 30, 31, 51, 71
Hill, George Washington, 71
Hilleboe, Dr. Herman E., quoted, 16
Hodgkin's disease, 81
Holders: cigarette, 33; filter, 55, 56
Horn, Dr. Daniel, 6; *see also* Hammond-Horn report
Hueper, Dr. W. C., quoted, 77
Hydrocarbons, 22-23
Hydrochloric acid, 46
Hypoglycemia, 48

Impotence, 2
Inhaling, 23, 34, 65, 66
Institute of Industrial Medicine, 22
International Cancer Congress, 23

Johnston, Dr. Lennox, 29; quoted, 58, 60
Jordan, Dr. Sara M., quoted, 47
Joules, Dr. Horace, quoted, 19, 37
Journal of the American Medical Association, 10; quoted, 18-19, 31, 35, 56

Korteweg, Dr. R., quoted, 17-18

Labeling, 75
Lancet, quoted, 58
Larynx: cancer of, 33, 41, 66, 77; Smoker's, 2, 10
Ledermann, Dr. Sully Charles Marcel, quoted, 79-80
Leukemia, 80, 81
Leukoplakia, 33
Levin, Dr. M. L., 31
Life Extension Examiners, 74
Lip cancer, 30, 31, 33, 34, 63, 66, 78
Lombard, Olive M., 62
Lung cancer, 41-44; causes of, other than smoking, 50-53; chances of developing, 2-3, 57, 67; death from, 1, 4, 7, 8, 11, 12, 15, 30; fear of, 54; in King George VI, 40; morbidity factor in, 49; in pipe and cigar smokers, 31, 32; prevention of, 81-82; primary lesions in, 10; reducing risks of, 65-67; research on, 22-24; statistical studies of, 13-19; surgery for, 1, 43, 44, 67; symptoms of, 41-42, 70; in women, 15, 25-26
Lymphomas, 80

Massachusetts Medical Society, 62
Maternal health, 27-28
Medical skepticism, 5, 18
Menstrual disturbance, 29
Metastases, 10, 44
Metropolitan Life Insurance Company, 52
Mice, research experiments on, 20-22, 32, 33
Micronite, 55
Milk of nursing mothers, nicotine in, 28
Minors, sale of cigarettes to, 75
Miscarriage, 29
Moore, Dr. George E., 33
Mouth: cancer of, 33, 34, 66, 78, 80, 81; holding smoke in, 66
Mucous membrane, 10, 46

National Cancer Institute, 16
Nervous system, 2, 47
New England Journal of Medicine, 5
Nicotine: addiction to, 58; amount of, in cigarettes, 55-56; in mother's milk and urine, 28
Nicotine amblyopia, 2, 48
Nicotine poisoning, 20-21
Norr, Roy, quoted, 68, 82
Nursing mothers, 28

Oberling, Dr., 17
Obstetrical patients, 27-28
Occupational disease, 51-52
Ochsner, Dr. Alton, 18, 19
Ogden, Dr. Henry Q., 25
Oral cancer, 33, 34, 66, 78, 80, 81
Osler, Sir William, quoted, 36, 80

Pasteur, 77
Perlman, Dr. H. H., 28
Pharynx, 2, 10
Pipe smoking, 30, 31-34, 63, 66

Pituitary gland hormones, 48
Postoperative complications, 11
Pott, Sir Percivall, 73
Prevention of cancer, 78-79, 81, 82
Preventive medicine, 76, 77
Primary lesion, 10
Proehl, Dr. Elsa C., 33
Pulse rate, 38

Radiation therapy, 81
Ray, Dr. C. J., 18
Reproduction, effect of smoking on, 28
Respiratory diseases, 2, 4, 5; *see also* Lung cancer
Rhoads, Dr. C. P., quoted, 16
Risks, reducing of, 65-67
Roffo, Dr. H., 23
Roth, Dr. Grace, 38, 56, 66
Rural incidence of cancer, 8, 24
Rush, Dr. Benjamin, 80

Scadding, Dr. J. G., quoted, 17, 30
Scrotum, cancer of, 73
Secondary lesions, 10
Sex, lung cancer and, 25-29, 52
Shoeneck, Dr. F. J., 28
Simmons, Dr. James Stevens, 77
Skin: cancers of, 21, 24; temperature of, 38, 39
Sloan-Kettering Institute, 16, 22-23
Smell, loss of sense of, 2
Smoker's Cancer (epidermoid), 12, 24, 26
Smoker's Cough, Throat, Larynx, Pharynx, Asthma. *See* Cough, Throat, *etc.*
Snegireff, Dr. Leonid S., 62
Sontag, L. W., 28
Sputum, cancer cells in, 42
Sterility, 2, 28
Stillbirth, 28
Stomach cancer, 46-47
Surgery, 1, 40, 43, 44, 67, 80, 81
Susceptibility, 3, 26-27, 64, 67
Sutton, Dr. John E., quoted, 37-38
Symptoms: of cancer, 41-42, 67, 70; withdrawal, 60-61

Taste, loss of sense of, 2
Temperatures: skin, 38, 39; smoke, 33
Testimonial advertising, 70, 75
Throat: cancer of, 31, 78; Smoker's, 2, 47
Thromboangiitis obliterans, 40, 41
Thrombosis, coronary, 36, 37
Tobacco chewing, 33, 80
Tobacco Industry Research Committee, 72, 74
Tongue cancer, 30, 31, 33, 66, 78

Ulcers, 46-47
Uranium miners, 50-51
Urban incidence of lung cancer, 8, 24, 51, 52-53
Urine: inhibition of secretion of, 48; nicotine excreted in, 28

Vocal cords, lesions on, 10

Withdrawal symptoms, 60-61
Women: lung cancer in, 15, 25-26, 52; pipe smoking by, 63; smoking by, 26-29; susceptibility of, to nicotine, 26-27
Wright, Dr. Irving S., quoted, 36
Wynder, Dr. E. L., 13, 20, 51, 52, 66; quoted, 32
Wynder-Graham report, 13-14, 25, 31, 32, 56

X ray, 43, 67, 80